SPIRITUAL MEDICINE

FOR

MODERN LIFESTYLE DISEASES

Dr. Dilip V. Kaundinya (MD)

SPIRITUAL MEDICINE
FOR
MODERN LIFESTYLE DISEASES

Dr. Dilip V. Kaundinya (MD)

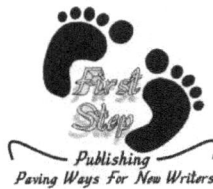

First Step
Publishing
Paving Ways For New Writers

First Published in 2019 by First Step Publishing

Editorial / Sales / Marketing Office at
303-304 Garnet Nirmal Lifestyles Ph 2
Behind Nirmal Lifestyles Mall
LBS Marg Mulund West
Mumbai 400080
E-Mail:- info@firststepcorp.com
www.firststepcorp.com

ISBN:- 978-93-83306-50-3
Price: India INR 275
Rest $15

Donation to World Renewal Spiritual Trust of
Brahma Kumaris, a NGO working for Global Peace,
Health and Brotherhood

God's formula for Success
Be Ever Ready, Ever Alert, Ever Attentive, & Ever Active
with a high Passion Quotient for
Your Set Goal

1. Watch Peace of Mind Channel 24 x 7
2. Visit the nearest BK Center for a Free of Cost Foundation Course
3. 11500 BK Centers Across 140 Countries
4. Make BK Rajayoga a part of Daily Routine
5. Phone : - 09999333555 / 666 for nearest center

Table of Contents

Foreword: Dr R. D. Lele

Science and Spirituality

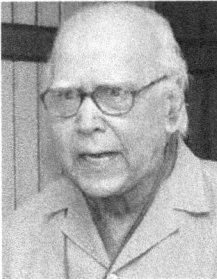

BY Dr. R.D.Lele, Padmabhushan, Padmashree, Dhanavantri award winner, Father of Nuclear Medicine in India, Present Director of Nuclear Medicine Division in prestigious Lilavati Hospital and Research Center, Mumbai.

MBBS [Osmania University], DTM & H [England], MRCP [Edin.], FRCP [London], FNAMS Hon., DSc Hon., Lit. Hon., Chief Physician and Director of Nuclear Medicine and Research & PET CT Dept., Jaslok Hospital and Research Centre,, Hon. Director of Nuclear Medicine and RIA Dept. Lilavati Hospital and Research Centre, Professor Emeritus of Medicine[for life] and Ex-Dean ,Grant Medical College and Sir J J Hospital, Mumbai. Dean [Academic], All India Institute of Diabetes, Mumbai. Emeritus Professor of The National Academy of Medical Sciences [India], Chairman Scientific Advisory Council, Haffkine Institute of Research, Training and Testing Centre, Mumbai.

The book "Spiritual Medicine for modern lifestyle diseases" by Professor D.V. Kaundinya falls in a rare category of books in Medicine. It deals with the

"Dis-eases" of the spirit [Atman] translating into physical ailments. All of them are associated with stress in mind. It tells about the value of incorporating spiritual medicine in modern therapies for the cure as well as prevention. An attempt has been made to explain the current scientific evidence behind healing by herbs in Charak Ayurveda and by Patanjali Kriya yog which includes yogic postures, Pranayam and meditation. Ancient methods of validating the findings were essentially "Experiential" i.e. based on "Experiences or Anubhav". A Chitta vrutti nirodh by meditation [Dhyan and Dharana] controls the agile mind and empowers it.

My views about the topic have been documented in my book entitled "Ayurveda and modern medicine [1986, second edition 2001]. However, the book by Professor Dr. D.V. Kaundinya opens up an opportunity for me to air them in detail. Ayurveda, a science of life, embodies ancient Indian experiential wisdom of over 3000 years. The Ayurveda concept of health includes body, mind and spirit [Atma]. Ayurveda prescribes "Swastha Vritta" fo maintenance of positive physical health and "Sada – vritta", ethical conduct for maintenance of positive mental health. Body, mind and soul are the trinity, the tripod. The life is the union of body, mind and spirit. Charak states- "harmonious and concordant interaction of body and mind causes "Well Being". The cause of disease, somatic or psychic, is either erroneous, absent or excessive interaction. Passion and delusion are pathogenic factors which are quietened by spiritual knowledge, philosophy and its practice in the form of fortitude, remembrance and concentration. There is great emphasis on mind control, "Chitta vrutti nirodh" and control of six enemies; "Shada ripus" like fear, anger, vanity, greed, jealousy and excessive attachment. He alone can remain healthy who regulates his diet, exercise and recreation, controls his sexual pleasures, who is just, generous, truthful and forgiving and who can get along with his kins. Just as the negative emotions of fear, hate, anger, greed, jealousy and frustration are life destroying; the positive emotions of love, hope, happiness, faith, confidence, creativity, will to live and let others live, will contribute to health and well being.

The Bible tells us that "A merry heart works like a doctor". Robert Burton, 400 years ago, in his "Anatomy of melancholy" emphasized the role of mirth and laughter as principle engines for battering the wall of melancholy and sufficient cure in itself. Sir William Osler regarded laughter as "Music of life" and that the people can keep themselves young with laughter. He also told that "Of the greatest duty of a physician is to teach his patients not take medicine." Dr. Norman Cousins [New England Journal of Medicine 1976] stressed the importance of mobilizing innate self healing power.

The limbic system has a "Pleasure centre" stimulation of which causes quasi-orgasmic bliss. And deep pleasurable relaxation mediated by encephalins, endorphins and cannabinoid [Anandamide, natural healers from the brain.]

Karl Popper has emphasized that science only tackles concepts which are testable, verifiable and falsifiable. The concept of heaven and hell is very attractive and has great utility for motivating the man to follow a "Straight Path", but it does not lend itself to scientific enquiry; so also the concept of karma, poorva karma and rebirth.

Twentieth century has made great strides in the study of human brain which is the organ of mind. The staggering complexity of human brain and its functioning is approached by "Cognitive Neuroscience."[Latin cognoscere, 'to know"]. A great deal about the mind has been learned from behaviour models of fitness in mental disorders. Further developments occurred through clinical observations, experimental paradigms developed in psychology and neuro-imaging, animal and human lesion studies of neural circuits, behavioural Neuropharmacology and Neuro-imaging. New technologies developed in last 30 years in cognitive Neuroscience including intra-transcranial magnetic stimulation [TMS], Magnetic encephalography [MEG], Functional MRI, Neuroreceptor imaging with PET and SPECT, have provided a wealth of information to mental processes— changes in blood flow in Depression, mood disorders and neuropsychosis, changes in regional neuro-receptors and neurotransmitter function [GABA, DOPAMINE, OPIOID, CANABIOID, SEROTONIN etc.] . The effect of BRAHMAKUMARIS RAJAYOGA MEDITATION was studied by Dr. Vikram Lele in 1987 along with Hertrhog of Zurich, Germany using FDH-PET CT [Fluorine -18-Deoxy Glucose] imaging showed a generalized hypo- metabolism related to

increased GABA activation, especially in the posterior regions of the brain EVEN WITH THE EYES OPEN. Interestingly two pegs of whisky produce the same effects. The Framingham study showed that those who jogged regularly for 45 minutes and took two pegs of whisky have the maximum longevity. But whisky may have serious side effects while with meditation there is no such risk. Hence I STRONLY RECOMMEND MEDITATION.

Professor Khetrapal at Lucknow used Functional MRI to study the effects of prayer and chanting of OM in various regions of the brain. Neural mechanisms of normal and abnormal cognitive processes in health and mental illness are now demonstrated by scientific approach. But the CONCEPT OF SOUL IS BEYOND THE CURRENT SCOPE OF SCIENCE and so also the concept of "Consciousness and Spirituality". To take a parallel in modern physics, NEUTRINO is a subatomic elementary particle with mass but no charge. Neutrino travels at a very fast speed and is currently the focus of intensive research worldwide. In India, Tata Institute of Fundamental Research [TIFR] Mumbai, VECC, Kolkata and advanced institute of Physics, Bhuvaneshwer have established the Indian Neutrino Observatory [INO], Madurai. I am tempted to speculate that by 2050, SPIRITUAL PHENOMENON could be explained in terms of NEUTRINO. Till that happens ONE SHOULD FULLY UTILIZE THE MESSAGE contained in the unique book of Professor Kaundinya.

In human motives, there is constant struggle between PREYAS, what one loves to do and SHREYAS-what is the right thing to do. Today the differentiation between these TWO PATHS in life is largely blurred and depends on a thin line. A finely tuned POWER OF DIFFERENTIATION acquired by meditation may help the humanity to pursue the morally and ethically RIGHT PATH IN LIFE.

14th September 2014

DR. R. D. LELE

Dr. Ramchandra Dattatraya Lele

Born on 16th January 1928 (Hyderabad city, AP)

Married July 1950, Wife Suneeta and 3 Children : Swati, Madhumati, Vikram

M.B.,B.S.(Osm.), DTM & H (Eng.), MRCP (Edin.), FRCP(London), FNAMS Hon. DSc., D. Litt

Fellow of National Academy of Medical Sciences, India

Founder Fellow of All India Institute of Diabetes

Founder Fellow of Indian College of Physicians

Colombo Plan Fellowship in Nuclear Medicine, Canada,1966 - 67

Former President of Society of Nuclear Medicine, India 1989

Former Editor-in-chief, Indian Journal of Nuclear Medicine,1990 - 96

First President, Indian Medical Informatics Association started in 1993

First President, Nuclear Cardiological Society of India started in 1994

First President, Society for Free Radial Research of India started in 2000

Member of Atomic Energy Regulatory Board, DAE, Govt. of India for 1990-2001.

Member of Editorial Board - Journal of Nuclear Medicine, USA - Journal of Nuclear Cardiology, USA

PRESENT POSITIONS :

Hon. Chief Physician & Director of Nuclear Medicine & Ex-Medical Director,

Jaslok Hospital & Research Centre, Mumbai.

Director of Nuclear Medicine and RIA dept., Lilavati Hospital & Research Centre, Mumbai

Emeritus Professor of Medicine (for life) and Ex - Dean Grant Medical College and Sir J. J. Group of Hospitals, Mumbai

Emeritus Professor: National Academy of Medical Sciences, India.

President, Independent Ethics Committee, India, started in 1999.

Member, Rotary Club of Bombay District 3140.

Chairman, Scientific Advisory Council, Haffkine Institute of Research, Training & Testing, Mumbai,

AWARDS:

- Received the Rotary Club's Distinguished Community Service award in 1990.
- 1st recipient of "Gifted Teacher Award" instituted by Association of Physicians of India, 1991
- Padma Bhushan Award, 1992 by the President of India
- Dhanvantari Award, 1997, by the Governor of Maharashtra State
- Hon. Degree of "Doctor of Science"- NTR University of Health Sciences, Andhra Pradesh, 2000

- Homi Bhabha Life time achievement award Indian Nuclear Society 2008.
- Prof. M. Vishwanathan National award of Excellence in Medical teaching & Medical Care, March 2012.
- D Litt. of the Chhattisgarh University of Life Sciences, 28th December2013.

BOOKS PUBLICATIONS: Over 100 Scientific papers and 9 Books

- Principles & Practices of Nuclear Medicine, 1984, Arnold Heinemann
- Ayurveda & Modern Medicine, 1986, Bharatiya Vidya Bhavan-2nd Edition 2001
- Computers in Medicine, 1988, 8th Reprint 1997, Tata McGraw Hill
- Medical Profession & the Law, 1992, 2nd Ed. 1993, Sajjan Sons
- Clinical Science & Clinical Research, 1993, 2nd ed. 2008 National Book Depot
- Rural Reconstruction: Challenges & Opportunities, 1996, Bharatiya Vidya Bhavan. This book is now available on-line in Million Book Digital Library Carnegie Melon, University Pittsburgh, USA
- Clinical Approach, 1997, Oxford University Press, Paperback ed. 2000, 2nd ed 2007 National Book Depot.

- Computers in Medicine: Progress in Medical Informatics: Tata McGraw Hill, January 2005. 3rd reprint 2009.
- Principles & Practice of Nuclear Medicine & Correlative Medical Imaging, 2009, Jaypee Brothers.

Foreword: Dr. Alaka Deshpande

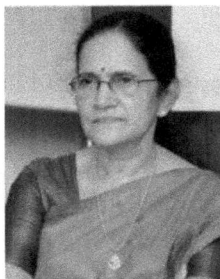

Health is defined as physical, mental, social and spiritual well-being.

The history of medicine reveals that primeval man with observations of the surrounding and with experience learnt to take care of his physical injuries. He then had no answer for microbial infections. He succumbed to tetanus, pneumonias and diarrheal diseases. Tuberculosis has been documented 3700 yrs. B.C.

Man's instinct for self-survival led to his quest for conquering microbes. He did achieve the success but microbes existing on this earth millions of years before the mankind proved smarter.

During the sojourn, the medical fraternity faced a new challenge of psycho-somatic disorders—somatic or physical manifestations due to deep rooted psychological problems. This was the beginning of a new discipline of psychiatric medicine. In Post renaissance era, the galloping growth in all the sciences resulted into technological advances in medicine. Many startling revelations made a better understanding of interplay of various neurotransmitters and their receptors. Molecular basis of disease pathogenesis started becoming apparent which helped to better understanding not only physical but mental disorders too.

However the concept and role of stress still remained ill understood.

New phenomenon of 'AFFLUENZA' has been identified after globalization which together with stress is the root cause of the present epidemic of life-style disorders like diabetes, hypertension and heart disease. They can be controlled but at present cannot be cured.
When the body is afflicted by such diseases how the mind can remain sound! The social health is affected by this evil or disordered mind !

Despite these amazing advances the birth and the death have still remained an Enigma !
Ray of hope comes from ancient scriptures of India! The Vedas have identified these disorders and elaborated the solutions. Ayurveda's principle is 'Swasthasya Swasth Rakshanam' i.e. maintenance of health by healthy lifestyle.

Vedas guide you to attain the spiritual health the ultimate goal of which is to conquer all the ailments for healthy mankind.

Prof Kaundinya, a microbiologist and a Rajyogi philosopher has very nicely explained the intricacies of the mind and body on the basis of various physical and chemical factors. He goes beyond it to the Spiritual Medicine.

The infinite energy of the Param Atman which imparts the life force energy to every living being can be experienced through Patanjali Yog-Sutra.
Dr. Kaundinya has opened a new vista for researchers to use newer techniques to explore unknown frontiers of the Spiritual Medicine!

I congratulate him and wish him all the success in his endeavours.

Padmshree Prof. Dr. Alaka Deshpande, M.D.
Consultant Physician, Former Prof & Head
Dept. of Medicine, Sir J J Gr. Of Hospitals, Mumbai

FOREWORD: Dr. Yusuf Matcheswalla

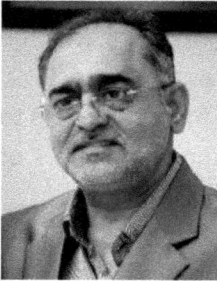

In today's world of rising Mental illnesses, depression, burn out, suicides, violence, rapes, addictions and exploitation of the needy by the greedy have become a common occurrence. Even the fun games have become a serious concern nowadays for example Selfie syndrome, internet addiction etc.

Scientism is an illness common in the learned and intelligent. This mind-set demands scientific proof for believing in God, The Supreme Father of all the souls. Dr. N.N. Wig, Professor emeritus of Psychiatry, PGI, Chandigarh, has labelled this state of mind as "Spiritual Vacuum." It leads to loss of differentiation between right and wrong. Here the right or wrong for all the human beings is defined by eternal universal cosmic laws of the Universe. All of the religious tenets are based on these fundamental laws of One and the Only One. Mind being nebulous and self-centred does not even think twice before manipulating even the tenets from God. Misinterpretation and forming a religious sub-sect is the consequence.

Holy Quran tells that a day shall come when whole of the mankind shall be disillusioned by the numerous religions and their sub-sects. That point of time, The Supreme selects a few who shall act as "Wahi" or Messengers. I have a reason to believe that Brahma Kumar's (BK) spreading the God's Message globally may be those Wahis. The main commandment in BK-organization is to attain a deity-like status by silent meditation and by the power of silence. The days before Kayamat in Islam and before final cataclysm in Hinduism describe the same scenario. Society ravaged by extremes of lust, violence, crimes, deceit and nepotism shall be evident.

Current studies in USA are proving that Tsunamis in human consciousness are producing the physical tsunamis of the world. It appears that the Devil shall succeed in his challenge given to All Merciful Allah the Supreme. Holy Quran took birth from the mystical experiences to Mohammad Paigamber. BK-tenets also came into existence in a similar fashion. Dada Lekhraj, an internationally renowned diamond merchant in Karachi got mystical experiences. Mohammad Paigamber is the last and the greatest of Messiah. But All Merciful Allah may have sent His Message through a minor and additional Messiah to save His beloved children from the ever tightening grip of Devil on the mindless humanity. Believers may choose the Right path or Sirat al mustaqim right now or it shall be never. It is also said that the non-believers shall enjoy a temporary prosperity and then they shall suffer for each of the crime they have committed. Two angels, one on shoulder are doing the job of recording each and every evil act.

Current advances in Psychiatry and Mind Body Medicine have shown that BDNF- Brain Derived Neurotropic Factor plays a key role in recovery from Depression. This book describes various drugs of God or rejuvenating neuro-hormones that are released from the brain during deep meditative states. Chapter on Novel instruments that demonstrate the deep meditative experiences is very relevant information in the context of Mind-Body Medicine. **But there is real need to evaluate and validate the results by these instruments Research in meditation** suffers because there is no uniformity in the definitions that were used for study. So results could not be compared scientifically. Experientially any meditation that quietens the mind and transforms the nature is the best panacea for the ills of the present times. The proposed definition mentioned in this book may be discussed for international uniformity in research. The new meaning to Mindfulness meditation given in this book liberates the mind from the firmly embedded concept that only Buddhist forms of Meditations are Mindfulness.

Mind empowerment techniques have evolved through Oedipus complex and Libido of Sigmund Freud, Psychotherapy of Gestalt, Psycho-synthesis and psycho-synergization of Robert Assagioli, Transactional Analysis

24

by Eric Berne and Rational Emotive Behaviour Therapy by Albert Ellis. Today Spiritually Augmented Cognitive Behavioural Therapy also has emerged. This book gives a very precise definition of soul, mind, intellect and traits. CQSE (Consciousness Quantum Spiritual Energy) is an extremely new concept about soul. Thought modulation for psycho-endocrine and immunological modulation is very interesting.

Time has now come when what Professor Kaundinya's proposed five emerging branches of the Mind-Body Medicine described in this book be given importance. And the knowledge of spiritual medicine should be included in MBBS syllabus for a meaningful research in various Institutes.

30-12-2017

DR. (PROF.) YUSUF ABDULLA MATCHESWALLA

Date of Birth: 04th August 1958
Nationality: Indian
Marital Status: Married
Address (Clinic): Masina Hospital Main Building,
1st Floor, Sant
Savta Marg, Byculla (East),
Mumbai – 400 027.

Address (Residence):   1603-A, Lady Ratan Tower,
Dianik Shivner Marg,
Off E Moses Road,
Gandhi Nagar, Worli
Mumbai 400 027
Mobile: 9820081884
E-mail: dryamatcheswalla@hotmail.com
MMC Registration No: 53949 (Maharashtra Medical Council)

EDUCATIONAL QUALIFICATIONS
M.B.B.S - 1983
Grant Medical College, University of Mumbai - Mumbai – India
M.C.P.S - 1983
Member of the College of Physician and Surgeons
M.D. (Psychiatry.) - 1988
Grant Medical College, University of Mumbai, Mumbai – India
F.I.P.S 1993

Fellow of the Indian Psychiatric Society

D.P.M (Diploma in Psychological Medicine) - 1991

College of Physicians & Surgeons-   Mumbai – India

M.D. (Forensic Medicine and Toxicology) - 1996

Grant Medical College, University of Mumbai - Mumbai – India

Post Graduate Diploma in Clinical Research – 2005

Institute of Clinical Research (India)

Post Graduate Diploma in Medico-legal Sciences - 2012

Symbiosis Institute of Management

F.A.P.A – 2010

Fellow of the American Psychiatric Association

Academic attachments (Teaching/Inspector/Research/Examiner/Quality advisor)

I.   Teaching

From 01st Jan 1991 to 10th November, 2007- Teaching General & Forensic Psychiatry to Undergraduate, Graduate & Postgraduate medical & nursing students at Grant Medical College & J.J. Group of Hospital

From 11th November, 2007 to date – Teaching psychiatry to nursing Students at Grant Medical College & J.J. Group of Hospital

From 15th February, 2006 to date Head of department & professor in psychiatry for course   Diplomate of the National Board (DNB), DPM (CPS) in Psychiatry at Masina Hospital, Mumbai

II.   Inspector – MCI   for Psychiatry Post Graduate Department from 2010.

III.   Research -Principle & co- investigator for 20 drug trials

IV.   Examiner

College of Physicians & Surgeons- MD Psychiatry

Narmad South Gujarat University- MD Psychiatry

Saurashtra University - MD Psychiatry

V.   Member -Quality Advisory Committee

Kishinchand Chellaram College of Science, Arts & Commerce - Mumbai

Professional Expertise

- General Psychiatry
- Emergency Psychiatry
- Child & Adolescent Psychiatry
- De-Addiction & Rehabilitation
- Geriatric Psychiatry
- Forensic Psychiatry
- Community Psychiatry
- Sexual Problems

CURRENT POSITIONS

Public Hospitals

- Honorary Psychiatrist & Honorary Associate Professor. - Grant Medical College & J.J. Group of Hospitals (Mumbai). (1994 till date)
- Honorary Psychiatrist and Head of the department Psychiatry unit II- Gokaldas Tejpal Hospital (Mumbai).(1997-2000) (2009 till date)

State Government

- Honorary Psychiatrist - Police Hospital (Mumbai)

Private – Charitable Hospital.

- Honorary Psychiatrist & Head of Department of Psychiatry - Masina Hospital
- Honorary Psychiatrist - Saifee Hospital (Mumbai)

Non government organization

- Chairman and Founder - Humanity Health Organization
- Chairman and Founder - Dilaasa - care givers support group
- Vice-President - Grant Medical College Student Association.
- Consultant Psychiatrist - Counselling & Suicide Prévention Centre (CASP).

Member

- Association of Medical Consultants, Mumbai
- E Ward Medical Practitioner Association, Mumbai
- A, C & D Wards Association
- Indian Association of Gerontology
- Indian Association of Occupational Health
- Grant Medical College Alumni Association
- Indian Society of Health Administrators

- Council of Sex Education & Parenthood

Past Positions
- Bombay Psychiatric Society (for 2006-2007)
- Indian Association of Child & Adolescent Mental Health
- Ex Deputy Coroner Mumbai - J.J Hospital from - 1996-98
- Governing Body Member   Indian Medical Association 2010-2011
- Chairman of Academy of Medical Specialties, IMA, Mumbai.
- Chairman Forensic Cell, Indian Psychiatric Society

Foreword: Dr Naras Bhat

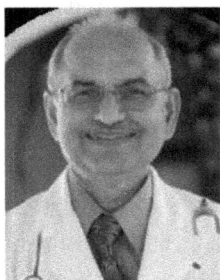

The book by Professor Kaundinya is a rare type of book which combines ancient Indian art and science of healing or yogic practices for health with the current research in Mind Body Medicine. The present materialistic world always wishes to know how to obtain quick and easy gains for whatever efforts they are taking. BK-Rajayoga technique and Total Health programme in the Appendix fulfils this essential requirement of the mankind. Pranayama Motivated Defecation for intractable constipation appears novel. But the claim needs to be substantiated by systematic research.

Stress is a major killer of the young today. My stress clinic practice is ten times more than the cardiology practice. My two books – Reversing stress and Burn out and how to prevent heart disease and cancer, have substantial reading clientele. The portable instrument RespErate mentioned in this book is extensively used in my stress clinic. Materialistic Americans usually do not know any relaxation or meditation techniques. So the instrument in my clinic has built-in music that relaxes the mind.

C.A.D. –regression by BK-Rajayoga in the publication by BK Dr. Satish Gupta could be tried not only in India but globally in different medical research institutes. Dean Ornish study is quite small and mainly based on strictly following the suggested lifestyle modification. Dr. Gupta's study is unique because the regular practice of BK-Rajayoga seems to confer the much needed self-determination that is required for following the suggested lifestyle modification for lifetime. In fact if a multi-centric research is undertaken and the claim is replicated, it could pave the way for a Health Policy aimed at substantial savings on stents and cardiac bypass in state Health budget. But India i.e. Bharat even today has a mental slavery which makes one believe that whatever is British or Foreign is good and better than our own. Doctors dismiss yogic and spiritual practices a blind faith or superstition.

Professor Kaundinya has given two very valid suggestions-

1] AYUSH should adopt any one school for a systematic research on Ayurveda and Yoga using ninth and tenth standard students who are extremely stressed out today. Health promotion by herbs and performance enhancement by BK-Rajayoga, Vipassana and Preksha Dhyan could be compared for results. This shall be the first step in establishing the value of AYUSH and Yoga in modern treatment and preventive strategies.

2] Various studies on meditation could not be compared because there is no uniformity in techniques used for meditation. Dr. Kaundinya proposes a composite definition of mindfulness definition for acceptance by the medical world. The effects of deep meditation and transcendence could be proved by ancient "Experiential evidence" used by Ayurveda to judge the efficacy of the drugs. But modern medicine demands scientific proof for the efficacy of the drug in pure form. Mainstream medicine forgets that a health promoting or disease curing herb has several components. Individually they may not have medicinal effect. But synergistically they become a powerful drug. Novel instruments described in the book could be used for two purposes- 1] to compare the results of various meditations and 2] for scientifically validating these instrument so that they become accepted for research purposes. The release of rejuvenating neuro-hormones during mindfulness and BRR −Biological Relaxation Response [Dr. Herbert Benson] needs to be investigated vigorously to prove the authenticity of the claims.

Spiritual Medicine for modern Lifestyle diseases is rare category of books which may motivate the common man to practice BK- Rajayoga or any mindfulness meditation that appeals to his mind for his health and problems. The postgraduate could take guidance from this book for a meaningful research in low cost or no cost asana, pranayama and meditation for health and cure. Sir J J Hospital, Mumbai is unique. It has a BK-meditation hut for the medical students and for the teaching faculty. The state of art chemiluminiscence machine in the Biochemistry department could be fruitfully employed for meditation research.

Five branches of Mind Body medicine or spiritual medicine open up numerous doors for a research which has a potential to receive global recognition immediately.

I hope if not all, at least Sir J J Hospital, Mumbai once more becomes a pioneer in global medical research. I congratulate Dr. Kaundinya for providing scientific proof for mysticism in spiritualism.

Dr. Naras Bhat
Professor of Mind Body Medicine
Seybrook University, Sanfrancisco USA
05-01-2018

○ ○ ○
SAMYAK DRISHTI

Dr. Sujal Shah
LASIK • Cataract • Cornea

Dr. (Mrs.) Manisha Shah
LASIK • Cataract • General Ophthalmology

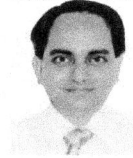

FOREWORD

Dr Sujal Shah

MBBS, DOMS, DNB (Ophth)

President-Jain Doctors Federation, Mumbai

This is a book about health and spirituality. A recurring thought in this book, is that religions and religious practices may be different, but, spirituality or the true spiritual philosophy is the same across all religions, if one can look beyond myopic pluralities. Ultimately, all religions were started by different spiritual seekers who attained self-realization or unity with their own consciousness and passed it down to their followers. Their preaching's in terms of practice may have varied according to their location and the prevailing times, or may even have been misinterpreted or distorted by their followers to create the differences apparent today. But, underlying in this diverse religious plurality is a common thread of spirituality i.e. Unity in Diversity. If we can learn to look at all human beings and by extension all life as having the same underlying consciousness as our own, our differences of religion, nationality, race, wealth, caste, creed and gender can easily be put aside.

Yoga is commonly interpreted as physical exercise today with accompanying health benefits. However, the word Yoga in its true sense in the Indian spiritual context means to join. Yogic practices help one to join the body with the mind and the soul. This book highlights the importance of yoga for physical and mental health refers to research in several institutes of Mind Body Medicine showing the benefits of Yoga in serious illnesses. Yoga too has many different schools to thought and differences in practice.

Dr Kaundinya candidly mentions his own experiences, wherein he was able to control several physical ailments by the practice of Bramhakumari Yoga, an apparently straight forward method of practising yoga to develop awareness of

101 / 202 A 1st / 2nd Floor, Sukh Sagar, N. S. Patkar Marg, Mumbai - 400 007.
Time : Mon. - Sat. 10am to 8pm • Tel : 2361 3937 / 2362 3937 • ☺ : 77382 73937
Mail : infosamyakdrishti@gmail.com • www.samyakdrishti.com
(Not for legal use)

Dr. Sujal Shah
LASIK • Cataract • Cornea

Dr. (Mrs.) Manisha Shah
LASIK • Cataract • General Ophthalmology

thought and action that sequentially gives physical, mental and ultimately spiritual benefits to the practitioner. He clarifies that Yoga is beyond the mere practices of asanas and pranayama. These are only the very beginning and the ultimate goal is a lofty one, that of attaining spiritual awareness and self realization.

Physical benefits and to some extent mental benefits are objective and can be demonstrated in a quantifiable manner. However, spiritual benefits of deep meditative techniques are experiential and may not be possible to demonstrate objectively. He argues, that the mere absence of proof is not tantamount to proof of absence. As a journey of a thousand miles must begin with a single step, initially research can focus on assessment of the physical and mental benefits of the regular practice of Yoga. At this time, because Consciousness itself is an enigma for modern science, it is likely that the spiritual benefits of Yoga will remain in the realm of subjective human experiences and will stay in the hearts, minds and spirits of Sadhak's who have attained them.

Following ones chosen school of Yoga can help the seeker to attain the heights he desires. Bramha Kumari Yoga of mindfulness meditation, according to Dr Kaundinya, is a straight forward approach that empowers the practitioner to focus on any single positive thought for any length of time and achieve tangible experiential milestones sooner than others. Having personally experienced some of the benefits of spirituality, he calls for the integration of Spiritual medicine in medical curricula.

There is no doubt Yoga is not a religion, it is a way of life. If we accept and embrace the fundamental concept of Yoga, the union of our body with our soul or consciousness and see everyone as manifestations of the same divine consciousness the physical, mental and spiritual problems that face us today will spontaneously fade away.

101 / 202 A 1st / 2nd Floor, Sukh Sagar, N. S. Patkar Marg, Mumbai - 400 007.
Time : Mon. - Sat. 10am to 8pm • Tel : 2361 3937 / 2362 3937 • © : 77382 73937
Mail : infosamyakdrishti@gmail.com • www.samyakdrishti.com
(Not for legal use)

Authors Heartfelt

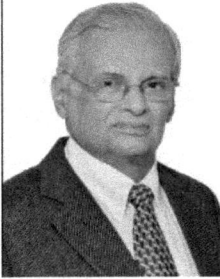

The main purpose of this book is to make the younger generation realize that ancient Patanjali sutra and Charak Sanhita are evidence based for health and performance enhancement. Dogmatism, divisionism, fanaticism and in the worst **case terrorism** are due to faulty interpretation of the tenets given in different religions. Spiritualism is a common thread that weaves through all the religions. Spiritualism and yogism are necessary for all human beings as the modern fast lifestyle has made the mankind to go against nature and lose the balance in all respects. **Internal balance is lost** giving loss of health, increased pollution and violence. **Global Consciousness Project** has proved that peace in the world could be restored by Mass Mind Intention using prayers and group meditation. **Tsunamis in mind result in the tsunamis of physical world.**

Quick burn out of the young and terrible addictions due to failures in life have become common. Balance between self- merit and expectations from life has been lost. Everybody wishes to own a Mercedes Benz. That is why spiritualism tells us that **all the desires are bad** as they give a restlessness syndrome till they are satisfied. Most funny part is that no sooner a desire is satisfied ,the second one immediately takes its place. **The culprit is the mind** which wants more and more. Patanjali Kriya yoga gives mind control [Mano-nigrah]. **Sleep-wake cycle** has been set against nature. Circadian bio-rhythms or Biological clock inside us has been set in accordance with sunrise and sunset since the origin of mankind. Our nocturnal habits have disturbed it so much that we require to learn "**Sleep hygiene**" merely to get a normal sound sleep. Sedatives become useless after some time. Ancient Vedas are actually scientific formula for leading our lives in accordance with unwritten but actually existing universal cosmic rules. **Laws of karma** are applicable to all human beings. Ignorance about them does not spare you from punishments. The horrific details of the punishment in proportion to Vikarma [Bad karma] are available in **Garud purana. Max Muller has said-** "There is no book in the world that is so thrilling, stirring and inspiring as the Upanishads.

German Physicist W. Heisenberg said-"After the conversations about Indian Philosophy, some of the ideas in Quantum Physics that had seemed crazy suddenly made much more sense." Current medical research highlights the value of asana, Pranayama, Dhyana and Dharana in health as well as man-management skills. **Ken Wilber's Transpersonal Psychology** talks about Atman to Atman transpersonal transactions for effective human resource management and development.

Spiritualism centres around metaphysical God and Atman or soul. Science has not been able to prove their existence. But that does not mean that these entities do not exist. Millions of people believe in their existence. **The definition of GOD** as Governing ,Operating, and Destroying and universally occupying benevolent healing energy becomes immediately acceptable to the **scientist minds**. But the Trinity of Brahma Vishnu and Mahesh immediately becomes labelled as **Indian mythology and myth**. God or Supreme Consciousness is the Supreme Creator, Operator and Destroyer Who creates the material world, provides energy to operate and maintain it and destroys whatever is evil or bad or effete and old. This super-duper scientist is running all the planets in all the galaxies in their pre-ordained orbits with **supreme accuracy** and without any exhaustible material fuel. No scientist till to this date has devised such a machinery. No wonder Sir Albert Einstein was made to say-"**Science is but an infant.**" Microcosm of Dr Deepak Chopra is a part and parcel of vast Universal or Cosmic consciousness. Human Being is a **BMSO- Body Mind Soul Organism**. Body is Humus or soil. It comes from soil and goes to the soil. **Being is existence**. Being is indestructible, immortal, ageless and disease less soul. **Wellness** comes only when Being is happy. Body consciousness today is so prevalent that the whole focus of drugs and cosmetics is only on the body. **Core personality is forgotten**. Bhagavad Gita tells that all the sufferings in life[Bhog] arise out of body consciousness. Therefore it advises to attain a **soul conscious state of mind**. BK-Rajayoga for me became a practical manual for attaining soul consciousness and thereby get liberation from all the troubles and problems in life. This **exhaustive author's heartfelt** is an attempt to convince the younger generation to include BK-Rajayoga in their daily routine and experience for themselves that they had discovered a **Kalpa vruksha** that fulfils all of their desires -materialistic as well as spiritualistic. **Split second Decisions** give the most accurate solution to the problems or difficult situations. Health comes automatically. Success becomes a foregone conclusion.

Core personality or Atman or sukshma sharir is of prime importance. But we neglect it. One soul several bodies in different births is true. **Past Life Regression Hypnosis and Therapy[PLRH& T]** provides the scientific proof. Body is a costume suitable to our role as an actor in this world drama. **Sanchit karma**[Prarabhda or Karmic Account] decides our costume, our role and the quality of life we have in this birth. Thus the health, happiness, harmony, peace and success in life is **pre-ordained** and occurs as per Divine script which we write with our own hands. BK-Rajayoga gives hope and optimistic solution that your **Bad karmic Load could be burnt out in Yogagni** or fire of yoga and tapasya. Tasting is the proof of pudding. I have experienced it.

Greatest folly a man today commits is that he presumes and assumes the **role of a Doer** while in reality he is just an instrument in the hands of the divinity. In BK-Rajayoga Atman plays the music in tune with divine commandments called as **Shrimat obtained at each Bk-centre through Muralis, a four page script** read in all 11500 BK-centres in 140 countries. Atman in tune with Shrimat performs a spiritual effort[**purusharth**] to attain a Personality of Excellence[**Purushottam**] or more precisely a Brahma type of personality. Charak Sanhita describes 15 types of personalities[prakriti] depending on the level of consciousness. There are three main levels of consciousness- **Satvik, Rajasik and Tamasik. Brahma type** is the highest, purest, most knowledgeful and most powerful among the

Satvik personalities. His soul is so powerful that it produces **a beneficial effect on the persons** in contact and purifies the whole atmosphere and nature with powerful and healing thought vibrations. Satanic or Asuri traits in the living beings get transformed into divine traits in a second. **Self-management and man-management** for such a person becomes very easy. He could mould others in accordance with his views. Success in any field becomes his birth right. **Vacha siddhi**, spoken words becoming a reality and **Sankalp siddhi**, the thoughts becoming an immediate reality becomes his usual and natural experience. The paintings of sages doing Tapasya and lions or tigers lolling harmlessly in front of them are not wild imagination but a scientific reality. Ever blissful state[**sat-chit-Anand** state] of consciousness manifests in his personality. Sthit-pragnya state of consciousness or a **state of spiritual equilibrium** becomes evident in such a personality. Grief and pleasure become equal to him in perception. There are eight levels of samadhi[**spiritual evolution**]. A level of 4 or above gives the power to materialize a golden Ganesh idol from thin air. Such super human powers are known as **Siddhis**. At seventh level beyond which eighth level **karmateet avastha** happens, a person comes to know the past, present and future in most precise and lucid terms. This is known as **Turia**

consciousness or Trikaal darshee avastha. This is because the microcosm becomes perpetually connected to a cosmic google called cosmic consciousness. Brahma type personality has **two divine qualities [Divya Guna]**- Tejas or glow over the face and Ojas or a soul level attraction for other souls. BK-concepts describe this state as **Roohe gulab** which gives a charisma to the person.

Siddhis even give the power of par-kaya pravesh, kaya-kalpa [rejuvenation to young form], levitation, clairvoyance and astral travel. A book entitled "**Kriya babaji and 18 Yoga siddhas**" by a Canadian, Marshal Govindan and "**Autobiography of a yogi**" by Swamy Yoganand Paramhans describe different siddhas and their miraculous powers. **Maha Avatar Nagraj Babaji** is the first disciple of sixteenth yoga siddha ,Sage Patanjali. One thousand years old Kriya babaji is still existing in the body of a 16 years old young person for the guidance of yogis beyond a certain stage of attainment. Adi Shankaracharya was the first disciple of Kriya Babaji. He wrote a wonderful poem. The gist of the poem told- " Strange was the sight that a 16 years old person, sitting under a Banyan tree and was teaching the aged disciples surrounding him. Still stranger was the fact that the whole transaction was taking place in total silence [without spoken words[**through thought**

vibrations]. The discovery of Mirror neurons proves that silent transpersonal human transactions are possible through thought vibrations. The reason for this Atman to Atman attraction or **Ojas** is the presence of mirror neurons in each one of us. The thought vibrations emanating from the soul forms the body aura which could be visualized by Kirlian Body aura photography. BK Dr Chandrashekhar, who recorded a miraculous recovery from a widely spread cancer by **Volcanic Rajayoga Meditation,** made an ingenuous use of Universal Scanner for showing the blocks in Energy Chakras and for recording the span of body aura. **Ojas is a divine quality** [Divya guna] that arises out of the presence of exceptional Right and Left Brain coherence as shown by EEG[Electro Encephalogram]. Such person also has unique and extra ordinary **empathy [samavedana]** for other persons. This Emotional Intelligence or a high EQ[Emotional Quotient] gives an uncanny ability to know by intuition where the other man's shoe is pinching. At the same time such person does try to remove this grief to the best of his ability and give immediate solace to the other person. Such quality creates a natural bonding between the two individuals. The persons then may risk even their lives to save such a philanthropic person. This is the most important quality in **a Leader without**

title. The people become his automatic and willing followers. Today in the higher posts of administration, Emotional Intelligence[EQ] is more valued than high Intelligence Quotient. Women have a natural and greater Right -Left brain coherence . No wonder they are the leaders who occupy high positions in almost every organization. Regular practice of BK-Rajayoga confers this increased coherence in men also. Emotional Intelligence is very important in man-management, Human Resource Development[HRD] and in **healthy doctor-patient relationship**. Development of just one divine quality shall reduce the incidence of court cases and assaults on the doctors. But Western medicine lacks a consciousness based approach and so doctors today have become money making machines in a majority of the cases. Greed has been ingrained in doctors as well as Pharma companies.

Magical advances in science and in the field of Artificial Intelligence **[AI]** has conferred miraculous improvement in Working Intelligence[WI] **of the robots**. But the best of scientists in the field of AI have not been able to inculcate Emotional Intelligence in the robots. These brilliant scientists frankly admit that their lack of understanding of the **phenomenon called as Consciousness** is responsible for this vital deficiency. Roger Sperry who got Nobel prize in 1970 for his concept of "One brain and two minds" tells that the Scientist mind in the dominant hemisphere is the root cause of the lack of Emotional Intelligence and most of the problems we face in this world. **This culprit mind** is judgemental about other persons and often finds faults in others. It self-centric and ego-driven. It wants to command and does not know how to mould. It is calculating and its relationships with other persons are based **on self-gains. It** likes to hear its own voice and often has a deaf ear for sound advice. It runs after higher and higher achievements often at the cost of others and its own health. **Winning in   Rat race** and cut throat competition against faith and religious and spiritual tenets bring positive outcomes for a short while. But soon they get replaced with stark failures. Their **self-centric** nature[vrutti] creates a negative impact on the workers underneath such persons. **Scientist Mind** is the seat of negativity. It is always full of negative thoughts like lust, anger, Ego, Greed, jealousy, hatred, doubt and repulsion. Today it is filled with stress, anxiety, tension, apprehension, fear worry and frustration out of its failure due to **comparison and competition** with others. Positive thoughts and healing emotions hardly ever arise in such a soul. It requires scientific proof before it can believe and have faith even in the God. Such persons firmly believe that they are self-made men forgetting that with such statements they relieve the Almighty of a terrible responsibility. **Spiritualist Mind** in the other hemisphere functions on belief, faith and positive thoughts and emotions. Philanthropy comes automatically to such persons. Spiritualist mind is the **sleeping giant** lying dormant in all of us. It has immense potential in terms of wisdom, experience and power. The experiences of past several births are stored in this mind. BK Rajayoga silences the internal noise in the Dominant hemisphere or Scientist Mind .This phase has been termed as Internal silence **[Antar mauna]** by the sages. The first and foremost quality this internal silence confers is an extraordinary ability of **Samyak shravana** [Holistic hearing] in which whole of the consciousness is focused on the act of listening. People could remember Veda by merely listening to them once [Ekpathy] because of this extra ordinary ability. The spiritualist Mind is a **super computer**. It tallies the present problem with the data of "Experiences" from the past several births and springs out a **solution almost instantaneously**. This is intuition or gut feeling or inner voice. The uncanny wisdom of going for an "**Extra mile**" comes from this mind. Out of world paintings and innovations come from this mind. Self-determination, self-discipline and self-dedication

47

for achieving a noble goal comes from this mind. This mind also gives a very meaningful **S.W.O.T. analysis**. It makes us realize our hidden potentials and strengths and also the weaknesses. Specific autosuggestions and visualization programme in Bk-Rajayoga removes the weaknesses and potentiate our strengths. Most important is that it confers an ability to differentiate between Opportunity and threat. Many times the threats in life come disguised as wonderful opportunity and the opportunity comes in the form of a threat. A wrong decision at this point of time means great loss or immense gain. Silence of Scientist Mind confers the ability to have an **accurate decision** in such matters. In spite of dominance of Scientist Mind first two seconds of silent transaction between the Mirror Neurons gives the most accurate judgement about the person or an event. This is the weak voice of Spiritualist Mind to help us. But in the **ever present ego** of a person makes him say " Let me think over it." Normally all the thinking is done by the dominant scientist mind. So even after a deliberate delay occurring because of thinking and having **second thoughts**, we take a wrong decision. This is known as **"Harding Error"** that may come in way of snap two second judgements by the Spiritualist Mind.. That is why intuition means listening to your inner voice with more care and attention. Harding error arises out of bodily charms of the other person. Person falls in love at first and then goes on repenting for whole of the life. Harding error is the root cause of divorces within six months of marriage in the younger generation today. Body consciousness brings the error in judgement though an Inner voice has protested.

Self-experience is the best teacher in the world. So here I shall elaborate the importance of BK-Rajayoga practice for health and self enhancement based on **my experiences** in life. I hope and trust that they shall form a **guiding beacon** for younger generation in the present turbulent times. A sharp Saraswat Mind, meritorious educational achievements and self confidence saw me becoming Professor and Head at a very early age of 31 years in Government institution. This was nothing less than a miracle for a Brahmin in reservation oriented system. So my natural conclusion was that I shall retire as the Director of Medical Education and Research. But **God had others plans for me**. So a very apt prayer should always tell God-" Please do not give me **what I desire**. But give me what You plan to give me in life because You know best what is best for me." Bhagavad Gita tells the same thing in different way-" Before time and above the fate no one gets in anything in life."

My posting at Swami Ramanand Teerth Rural Medical College at Taluka place called Ambejogai in the most backward Beed District was the turning point. A **phase of intense problems** began. I was promoted to the post of Professor and Head in 1981. But malignant cast politics of unimaginable intensity made me a victim. An acting and most corrupt Dean of a particular powerful category facing numerous enquiries due to gross financial irregularities, wrote adverse CRs out of jealousy and fear that I may rob his post. He went on taking out his venom for nine years. **This was against rules. Adverse CRs have to be communicated in the same year so that one gets adequate notice** to show improvement. The result in 1992 was that I was demoted to the post of Associate Professor on which I was promoted by MPSC selection **in 1973**. Once again Divinity intervened. A Matt judgement and efforts of **Late Gopinath Mundeji and Pramodji** reversed the reverses immediately so that I remained a Professor with a proverbial Damocles' sword of demotion and transfer hanging over my head. The complete justice was done in **1996 killing all of my chances even to become a Dean**. Thus I missed becoming the Director. BK-concepts and also Bhagavad Gita tell us that "Every moment of the word drama is most accurate and most beneficial. Whatever has happened is good.

Whatever that is happening is better and whatever shall that happen in future shall be the best." At that point of time it was difficult for me to swallow this **spiritual wisdom**. My mind kept on asking – **"Why me"?** Retrospectively when I introspect , I realized that every word of wisdom was accurately correct. Had I been promoted as the Director, I would have spent all the remainder of my service kissing the feet of greedy politicians. The **quantum jump in the Quality of Life** I am experiencing after adopting BK-Rajayoga in my daily routine, would never would have come my way. I must narrate some more incidences to prove my point. A transfer from **rural medical college** to advanced tertiary care hospital in **Mumbai** would have devasted many lesser souls. Brain of a Saraswat gave me the fame as examiner who asks tricky and very meaningful questions. At the same time generosity which probably I developed in **the Sangam Yug[Era of confluence]** of previous birth kept me generous with marks. In fact I used to assure each and everybody that your passing marks you have already earned by your mere presence. Answers to questions shall differentiate a distinction holder. **Dr Mrs Kaundinya ,Professor and Head of Physiology, was most popular amongst students as her teaching made** the subject very easy. Students' feedback always told that Microbiology and Physiology are the best departments in teaching. At one of point of time there were as many as **14 distinctions is Microbiology**. In our times Distinctions were rare and exceptionally brilliant person used to get it. So a question arose- Are the students so brilliant or our teaching is out of this world? My mind told me that these two could be contributing factors. **But real performer** is MUHS pattern of examinations with **MCQ, BAQ, SAQ and set of FAQs**[Multiple choice questions, Brief Answer Questions, Short answer questions and Frequently asked questions.] In short it was made very difficult for the student to fail. At the same time setting of the question paper became an **ordeal for the examiners**. Many appointed their juniors privately for such onerous tasks and of course with nothing more than good will which helped in postgraduate examinations. **Dr Dongaokar the first VC** took lifelong and more than adequate revenge over the examiners and medical teachers. The vacations also became reduced to half. **A hell has been created for the medical teachers** and the examiners. Slightest mistake in filling the complicated mark sheets became an offense under **UNFAIR MEANS** and the poor examiner has to report to Nasik at his own expenses like a **hardened criminal reporting to police station where the clerks donned role of a judge**. At MUHS after a wait of several hours revelation used to come that a countersignature was required on a particular page. **Not a single Vice chancellor has made an effort to change the harassing rules for the examiners and a paltry sum as remuneration**. BK Rajayoga gave such mind empowerment that I did not have to face any such ordeals because of the focus.

Immense stress gave me seven incurable diseases ranging from chronic cough, cervical spondylitis, Thyrotoxicosis, Chronic fatigue, severe back pain due to Spondylolisthesis, tendoachilles tear while practising for veteran tournament and almost a burn out. **Bk-Rajayoga gave impossible and permanent cures.**

Saraswats are God fearing and highly superstitious. BK-Rajayoga gave **emancipation** from several false beliefs and superstition. One of these I must mention. I used to worry on two counts while on the Path of Bhakti.

1] I used to fear that my non-vegetarian food habits surely shall give me a birth in the Yoni of a tiger. Once that happens how I shall hope to become grass eating tiger? Otherwise how I could come back to **human yoni?**

2] Secondly everybody these days is telling that **kayamat or Pralaya** or final deluge is very nearby. How painful it shall be to die by drowning?

Muralis which are from mystical experiences to a human conduit Brahma Baba removed these major fears. God Himself assured that a human being always takes the birth of a human being. Secondly, India i.e. Bharat never goes under the water as Incorporeal God Shiva always takes Avataran only in Bharat.

Another most assuring part was that God assured repeatedly in His Muralis that He will move with a protective umbrella over your head provided you always remain busy in His remembrance. The **Yogagni** [Fire of Meditation] shall burn out all of your Bad karmic Load and emancipate you from pain and suffering. I have several personal experiences about these novel guarantees by the Supreme Father of all the souls.

The "Experiences" and divine Muralis helped to set an **elevated goal for myself**. Geriatric OPD in Sir J J Hospital revealed to me the End stage battle of the soul before final emancipation as a consequence of unfinished Karmic Load. The visits to old age homes revealed **the hell** that awaits us if we do not shed our bad Karmic load by intense spiritual effort[**Purusharth].**

Interactions with **AYUSH and NCD wing** of Director of Health Services since **2012** revealed the horrible plight of doctors and of everybody in this horrible era called as Iron age[Kali yug] due to stress born NCDs[Non-infectious Chronic Diseases]. **NCDs are non-stop CDs of pain and sufferings**. They include diseases ranging from Obesity, acidity, insomnia , Diabetes, Depression and Heart attacks to cancers, Parkinsonism and Dementia. Suicides, Burn out and addictions are the common consequences. Sometimes the pain and suffering is so intense that there is a cry for **euthanasia or mercy killing.**

Another very serious problem is that noble healthcare profession has become **five star sickness care Industry.** Firstly fall ill and then we shall take care of you at an astronomical cost of course to compensate for our troubles. Falling ill has become a crime for a common man because his illness may devastate the family financially and permanently. No wonder an exodus has begun towards Complimentary Alternative Medicine[**CAM]** which are beyond any control like that by FDA. So several unfortunate people are becoming **victims of quackery**. Modern Medicine promptly declares all such modalities of treatment as " **Pseudoscience" without** making any effort to test the claims of cure by CAMs.

My "experiences" with BK-Rajayoga gave me firm belief that "**An awakening** " of both the doctors and the common man is necessary to make Bk-Rajayoga as evidence based panacea for all illnesses. BK- Rajayoga is an easy meditation for very busy people today.So Divine Plan made me the chairman of a novel MUHS committee to include "**Ethics and Spiritual Medicine in MBBS syllabus" in the year 2013.**

First problem was the absence of a book that gives consciousness based approach to health and cure- which modern medicine calls as **The Whole Person Medicine**. Supreme Teacher got a book entitled "**Spiritual Medicine for modern lifestyle diseases,**" written by me in the year 2013 itself in mere 21 days while at Bengaluru. This book then went through obstacle race from 2013 to 2018 for getting published. Funny part was that the whole of medical wing of Brahma kumaris felt that my book is not worth publishing by the BK-Literature department. But a **miraculous Divine plan** reached the book to all the International BK-Centres due to **BK Amola Shah of Florida**. Second edition is now getting published by **First Step Publishers in 2019**. A review of the book appeared in Antiseptic Journal in **December 2018.**In the same month, review article entitled – "Meditation versus Relaxation" by myself and Dr Mrs. S. D. Kaundinya got published in the International Journal of Basic and APPLIED Physiology. All of these are miracles in accordance with a Divine script.

Now the next target was to prepare a **short add-on syllabus in spiritual medicine so that MCI permission should not become necessary.** Syllabus submitted in May 2013 became modified to mere **five lectures and five "Experiential sessions"** to be conducted only in the first Academic term of three subjects- **Physiology** at First MBBS level, **Forensic Medicine** at Second MBBS level and **General Medicine** at Final MBBS level. Every care was taken so that the syllabus should not be a burden to the students. Secondly the medical students shall have a prolonged and perpetual exposure for the entire tenure in a medical college of four and half years, to three evidence based mindfulness meditation-

1] Vipassana of Buddhism 2] Preksha Dhyana of Jainism and 3] BK-Rajayoga. The students shall be able to decide which meditation suits them best for their stress management and performance enhancement. Present VC Dr Dileep Mhaisekar had put up the syllabus for discussion in Academic Council in **June 2017. But medically illiterate majority did not allow the VC to implement the recommendations at MUHS level and forced him**

to submit it to MCI for permission. Today MCI stands dissolved.

A fresh struggle to implement the syllabus in spiritual Medicine began **in 2019**. The following eminent personalities in the field of medicine have given the foreword for my book-
1] Padma Bhushan **Dr R. D. Lele,** Director of the division of Nuclear medicine, 2]Padmashree **Dr Alaka Deshpande** Professor and Head of Medicine and central Nodal officer for AIDS control 3] **Dr Yusuf Matcheswala** Honorary Professor of Psychiatry at Sir J J Hospital , Mumbai 4] **Dr Naras Bhat**, Professor of Mind Body Medicine , Seybrook University, Sanfrancisco, USA and 5] **Dr Sujal Shah** a renowned Retinal specialist and the President of Jain Doctors" Federation. All of them sent letters to Honourable Academic Council of MUHS recommending the acute need of including Spiritual Medicine in MBBS syllabus. They have pointed out that **USA** has started undergraduate and post graduate courses in Spiritual Medicine in the year 2001 itself soon after **WHO** added spiritual health in its definition of total Health in the year 1998. Other developed countries have followed USA. But India ie Bharat

Is minimum of 18 years behind the world. A great Nation which made the whole world celebrate **International Yoga day on every 21st June** is so much behind in implementing a thoughtful recommendation for bringing a better tomorrow in the present Health scenario, is both **shameful and retrogressive.**

Another very pertinent fact is that the demand for teaching and training in spiritual medicine has been ascertained from the medical students and the specialists by **two CMEs on " Value of spiritual and yogic strategies in modern medicine"** in Sir J J Hospital, Mumbai held in January 2014 and March 2014. Both the KAP study [Knowledge Aptitude and Practice] and Feedback study on two CMEs have been published in medical journal.

A majority [98 per cent] of participants opined as under-

1] They know that spiritual and yogic practices are necessary for their health and stress management. But they are in absolute confusion. There are multiple yoga systems and each one tells it is the best amongst all. Many come in commercial packages. So the mind is unable to decide.

2] They shall never depend upon non-medical self-**proclaimed spiritual Gurus** to learn Yogic practices. They shall always prefer teaching and training by a trained member of teaching Faculty. **Such Faculty which has official recognition could only be created once the spiritual medicine gets incorporated in MBBS syllabus.**

If **Dr Mhaisekar** succeeds in his ceaseless efforts then MUHS shall be the first Medical University in India which has followed USA and other advanced countries in bringing the syllabus to **global standards**. **NCD wing** shall have adequately trained doctors to apply meditation as therapeutic strategy. Alarming rise of NCDs in young population shall be checked and may be eradicated. Health Budget of Maharashtra could be drastically reduced. My dream of "My India, Healthy, Happy and addiction free India" shall become a reality.

Robin Sharma has given excellent recipe for success in life in his two very wonderful books.. But they become practical and applicable only if person has an empowered mind **and** health by regular practice of BK-Rajayoga. The book "The monk who sold his Ferrari" describes an American advocate who was busy enjoying everything fast in his life. One day he collapses in the court room with massive heart attack. His doctor gave him two alternatives- "Leave the practice to live well or continue with the practice and drop dead eventually." The advocate wanted to go to Himalayas .So he sold his practice to his assistant. The first chapter begins with the assistant burning the midnight oil when a 30 years old person forcefully enters his chamber. The assistant mistook this person to be the son of his former employer. As it turned out the former employer himself was standing before him. I am sure this kaya kalpa[Magical rejuvenation] has happened because of the kriya yoga that sages in Himalaya taught him. Robin Sharma has not elaborated on this aspect. The second book gives magical formulae for success in life by discovering a leader sleeping silently in all of us. But I believe that these formulae shall never succeed in bringing out the desired transformation unless and until help of daily BK-Rajayoga is taken. The much needed self-determination, self -dedication and self- discipline comes only sadhana of BK Rajayoga.

12 March 2019
Dr D.V. Kaundinya MD

Magic of Modern Medicine Vanished

Anything that is secret and mysterious in the various systems of yoga should be at once rejected. The best guide in life is strength. In religion as in all other matters, discard everything that weakens you. You should have nothing to do with it.

- *Swami Vivekananda*

Historical landmarks reveal that the modern medicine is only 400 years old. Antibiotic era and the era of chemotherapy of infections began with the discovery of Penicillin in 1928. The miracle happened in a policeman with severe staphylococcal infection. So penicillin was nicknamed as "magic bullet." Infections were controlled. Immunology began with Jennerian vaccination. [1-Dey] Vaccines, toxoids and antiserum against microbial infections and for cancer became available. But soon Nature bowled another googly. Auto-antibodies against the self-antigens gave intractable autoimmune diseases. Viral diseases brought fresh headaches. Anything that could not be diagnosed became viral fever. Discovery of anti-viral drugs brought in a novel syndrome of AIDS followed by Ebola haemorrhagic fever, H1N1 and air-borne Zica virus. Dr. Hegade former Vice Chancellor of Manipal University tells in scientific seminars that both H-1N1 and Zica virus are the brainchild of greedy pharma companies. Conventional and rational medicine became a controversial expensive healthcare Industry aimed at exploitation.

Somewhere in the journey of oppression and killing by powerful antibiotics, super bugs emerged in revolt. An Australian Olympic swimmer was about to get his hand amputed because of the infection by a super bug against which no antibiotic is available today. Divine Grace intervened and the hand was saved from amputation. The World Health Organization made antimicrobial resistance the theme of the World health day of the year 2011.The WHO representative to India, Nata Menabde spoke to TOI. She told that the arsenal to fight microbes is very weak right now. Antibiotic resistance is a very serious problem. It endangers human lives when the antibiotics don't work.

Stress became a cause of incurable lifelong diseases roughly from 1994[Sheridan 2]. Today stress associated diseases are known as NCDs- Non-infectious Chronic Diseases. Alarming rise in NCDs forced Directorate of Health Services to open an independent wing in 2012 to tackle this global menace of Diabetes, Dementia, Depression, cancer, heart attacks and degenerative diseases. Paradoxical rise in incidence of NCDs continues because the current generation of Indian doctors do not have the knowledge of Spiritual medicine and evidence based yogic techniques for cure and prevention. Two latest branches of Medicine called as Energy Medicine and Mind Body Medicine made their appearance. Collectively they are known as Spiritual Medicine. Prana became known as Life force energy and consciousness based eastern approach to medicine became applied. Whole Person Medicine of 1000 years old Charak sanhita became a current medical jargon in USA[3- Avadesh Sharma].

Mind Body Medicine presently has five branches-
1. Psycho-neuro-endocrinal immunology [PNI]
2. Psycho-oncology [Carl Simonton]
3. Psycho-pharmacology- Placebos have become 70 to 300 times stronger than disease specific medicine.
4. Neurogenetics – Allen's Brain map and dangerous cerebral genes.
5. Ken Wilber's Transpersonal Psychology - Human Resource Development [HRD]

All of these developments have their origin in ancient systems of healthcare like Charak's Ayurveda, Unani, Homeopathy and other complementary alternative therapies. [CAM]. **But Machiavellian** Thomas Babington Macaulay   cleverly programmed the brilliant Indian minds in such a way that even today Indians believe that whatever is British or foreign is good and greater than our own.
[4- Hegade-2008]

Indians have forgotten their brilliance of mind which could remember Vedas merely by listening to them. Samyak shravan in Buddhism means whole consciousness should be focussed in the single act of hearing. This ancient art is lost. Persons today mainly listen to the inner din produced by a storm of negative thoughts and emotions. Ancient Indian wisdom calls them as Vikalpa, Vikara, Vasana and Vikshepa. Looking at a person or event through the goggle of previous or past experiences gives a grossly distorted perception. This is famously known as 'Goggle effect' or vikshepa.

Vedanta indicates a phase in the eternal Time cycle or world drama when soul and mind power became so diminished that Vedas became beyond the understanding of human intelligence. Mystical experiences to sage Patanjali gave Kriya yog to the mankind for emancipation from pain and suffering [5 – Taimini 1961, 6, 7]. This Ashtang yog or Indian Integral Yog promises conquest of grey hair, dim vision ageing and diseases. Pranayama, Dhyan and Dharana enhance life force energy. Thus obvious inference could be that total health according to the definition of by WHO [1998] could be directly linked with mind power or soul power and life force energy. Please note that there is no mention of any God in Kriya yoga. Seventy years old Ramdeo baba could be taken as the living example for the claim of conquest of ageing and greying by Kriya yog. A person who was a non-entity has become world famous for his "Message" about yoga for health. In the process he became a latent force behind the million dollars industry and also a powerful motivator for common man adopting yoga in his daily routine [Dincharya]. Is this not a divine miracle? Young generation half the age of this extra-ordinary Yogi seek costly hair transplant procedure for their baldness.

Patanjali was the sixteenth amongst the eighteen yoga-siddhas. [6- Marshal Govindan].All of them possessed super human powers like clairvoyance, levitation, power to walk on fire or water, astral travel, par-kaya-pravesh, suspended animation and the power to convert any metal into gold [alchemy]. They studied human anatomy and Physiology by taking their consciousness inwards.[6].The life details with photographs of all the yoga-siddhas are available except for the first yoga-siddha known as Shiva. This is probably an indirect proof about the incorporeal God Shiva who gives mystical experiences to the chosen human conduit for transmitting a "Message" that shall ensure health, happiness, harmony and peace.

Boganthar, the first amongst yoga-siddhas went to China to liberate the people there from sufferings by his acupressure and acupuncture techniques probably because of the mystical experiences given to him by incorporeal God, Shiva

Today these ancient techniques fall in the category of Energy Medicine. In China, at some place, the statue of Boganthar bearing his Chinese name is present and being worshipped by the locals [6]. Korean spiral therapy a form of acupuncture therapy is believed to have cured cricketer Yuvraj of his malady and Sania Mirza of her severe shoulder pain after the operation. [TOI 20-th October 2008]. These are the incidences where modern therapy has not given desirable results. But Indian Macaulay programmed mind crosses all the limits of rational scepticism. [TOI- news]. Criticism without any scientific validation is futile. Instead a systematic research needs to be done in various prestigious research institutes about the claims of miraculous cures. The scientifically proved complementary alternative therapies then shall save the mankind from exploitation. Unfortunate patients with end stage disease like cancer or AIDS become an easy prey to exploitation.

Radionics[Mumbai], Prolo-ozone therapy at Mount Abu and Cytotrone therapy at Bengaluru are a form of energy medicine which have saved several knees from expensive replacement. But a rigid mind-set of modern medicine takes pleasure in refusing to believe without taking trouble of disproving the claim by systematic research. Kinsel and Strauss 2003[8] have recorded that a rigorous research is needed to support claims by Complementary Alternative Therapies[CAM].

Current research in several Institutes of mind body medicine in USA have proved that yogic postures, pranayama , Dhyan and Dharana have great potential in maintaining the health ; and also for the cure and rehabilitation in various diseases[8- Bijalani 2011 and 9-Best & Taylor 2012]. Sirtuins secreted during Mindfulness meditation retard and reverse ageing [10-Naras Bhatt,11- Jay Quinalan].

Single pointed focus of thoughts [6- Ekagra chitta avastha –Sage Patanjali] empowers the mind by raising the consciousness from basal and harmful Rajasik-Tamasik state to an elevated and powerful Satvik or soul-conscious state. Empowered mind then is able to avoid falling in honey-trap or money trap set by devil and is able to guide a person on the straight path, Sirat al mustaqim or path of shreyas. There are eight levels of spiritual evolution [12 – Chinamaynand 1984, Mandukya Upanishad]. The highest and most powerful and pure state of consciousness is known as Brahma type [3-Avadesh Sharma 2009]. This Turia consciousness gives the power to perceive the past, present and future in very precise terms.[Trikaal-darshi avastha.] The ancient term consciousness, even today, remains an enigma to the brilliant scientists in the West who have brought miracles in the working intelligence of the Robots. It is for this reason that they are not able to introduce emotional intelligence in their creation.

Gene therapy, cloning, stem cell therapy and several others promised a lot. But they failed miserably within a short time to provide lasting cures. Stress, an omnipresent and omnipotent killer of the young today arises in mind. Mental disorders also have their origin in mind or manamaya kosh [12 Chinamaynand-Charak sanhita]. But a clear cut definition of mind is not available in modern medicine. Secondly action of all the drugs even those used in psychiatry is limited to superficial most Annamaya kosh. Even the five body sheaths surrounding the core personality of Atman is not known to modern medicine. Naturally N.C.D. wing opened in 2012 is only recording the rise in cancers and other such incurable NCDs. Cancers have recorded 45% rise in incidence. Heart attacks have become common even in young cardiologists. Every third Indian today is Diabetic and Hypertensive. That means millions that were spent on celebrating Hypertension day, Heart day or Diabetes day have gone down the drain. Current scourge of mindless violence, road rage, satanic and cruel rapes, addictions, Burn outs, suicides, fatal attraction called, Selfie-syndrome obesity, insomnia and degenerative diseases show the grossly visible signs of the failure to control NCDs. AIDs also arise in Mind as an aberrant thought and a mindless immoral act. HIV comes much later in the picture. But do we have any mind modulating technique? Dhyan and Dharana are now evidence based thought transformation and mind modulation techiniques. Unfortunately in India nobody believes and has faith in the ancient Indian art and science of healing in the form of Charak's Ayurveda and Patanjali Kriya yog. Even a stubborn mind-set is an ego driven aberrant mind-set [Vrutti]. No wonder we Indians do not remember what 5000 years old

Bhagavad Gita has told- "Our thought forms the seed of our karma and destiny." Western psychiatrists today, believe that this ancient scripture is the most powerful book on psychotherapy and Arjuna to be the first case of depression. [3- Avadesh Sharma].

Transferring of Cosmic healing energy by a pranik healer cures various diseases which have been declared as incurable by modern medicine. Dr. Mulk Raj Dass at Musoorie [Deccan Herald 15-02-2009] is a famous pranik healer. Even Chronic Hepatitis and paralytic patients showed cure by their medical reports after the therapy at the camp. Dr. Dass had worked as a scientist at Max-Planck Research Institute at Berlin. Dr. Dass tells that in 1997 he discovered the power of his touch and miraculous ability to heal quite coincidently. He bandaged his colleague and the colleague discovered that his pain has mysteriously disappeared. Dr. Dass came to Musoorie to mitigate the suffering of masses in India. He says that despite being a scientist he failed to find a concrete definition of the therapy. METAPHYSICAL entities always pose this dilemma for the modern doctors.

Today a man has come to know that controlling one's mind is the best solution to all of social and health problems he is facing. But powerfully negative atmosphere has made agile mind totally out of control of a human being. Today 90% of the children suffer from ADHD- Attention Deficiency Hyperactive Disease.

Both parents and the patient prefer therapy by group meditation over that by drugs. A large majority of these children retain their disease in their adulthood. Such adults get bored very quickly. So they go on leaving their jobs at the drop of a hat. Soon jobs do not come their way. A suicide or a Burn Out is the dreadful result. Seeking pleasure from anything new becomes their lifestyle. Result is sexual aberrations, addictions and shopping binge. Selfie syndrome, a novelty soon became a deadly craze. Healthiesm or Jolie syndrome is another example. Risk of surgery for breast removal is preferred over a possible cancer in future. Psycho-oncology utilizing healing power of mind harnessed by meditation is never considered as a choice. So Dr. N.N. Wig , Professor emeritus of Psychiatry, PGI, Chandigarh, came out with a mental affliction now known as Spiritual Vacuum.[3- Avadesh Sharma]. Spiritual vacuum leads to loss of power of differentiation. Person then pursues a wrong, unethical and immoral Path and begins his slow muffled march to the grave in intense pain and sufferings. Bhagavad Gita calls these physical and mental pains as Bhog. Spiritual Health on the other hand ensures a life full of Energy, Enthusiasm and happiness [High EEH value] till the last breath.

Dr. Richard Davidson [13] Professor and Head of Psychiatry, Wisconsin University, in 2003, coined the term Mindfulness Meditation for ancient Dhyan and Dharana. Since Dr Davidson worked with Vipassana, the term Mindfulness became synonymous with Buddhist form of meditation. **Author proposes an all-inclusive definition of Mindfulness.** It is an ability of having a controlling and ruling power over the agile mind of such magnitude that one is able to stabilize it on the present moment or a single positive thought at any time and for any length of time.

Calm and stress free mind is very important for health. Dr. David Eddie [4] Professor of cardiac surgery used his Archimedes model to assess the effect of modern therapies in increasing the lifespan. This virtual model had all the physiological and Biochemical parameters that are functional in a human being. Results were startling. Trillions and trillions of dollars spent on expensive interventions increased the life span by mere 3 per cent. Rest 97% came from proper sanitation, proper nutrition, proper sleep and a tranquil state of Mind. Mindfulness meditative techniques ensure a calm mind under any adverse event or circumstances. Sleep back log today has now become potential health hazard. Sleep hygiene has come into fashion. BK-Rajayoga provides tangible solutions to the problems of sleep and jet lag.

A central Government enterprise, AYUSH – Ayurveda, Yoga, Unani, Siddha yog and Homeopathy could undertake a systematic research for Health promotion, Intellect enhancement and mind empowerment by application of ancient Ayurvedic system of herbs and meditation by adopting any one of the schools. This shall go a long way in removing the belief in modern mainstream medicine that these modalities of therapy are superstition or blind faith or unscientific quackery. The state of art equipment in Sir J J Hospital, Mumbai could assess the level of health promotion and stress management by herbs and meditation. This effort shall add a new and meaningful dimension to the celebration of International Yog day of 21st June every year. Not long ago, Charak had described herbs for complete rejuvenation or kaya kalpa.

Author by using the God given quality of perseverance has been able to initiate BK-Rajayoga sessions for the parents and the students of ninth and tenth standard in the local Arunodaya School at Thane because of a proactive Principal, Mrs Shilpa Jejurkar with effect from January 2018. Dr. Kiran Pandit, an Ayurveda specialist having his own hospital, on behalf of AYUSH has promised to initiate a research using Buddhivardhak herbs in a one year project. The results shall give a composite evidence based report about the herbs for health and wisdom and mind empowerment by BK-Rajayoga.

Whole hearted co-operation and involvement from the Directorate of AYUSH, Health Services in Maharashtra and the Directorate of Medical education and research shall certainly bring a better tomorrow in the present health scenario.

An add-on syllabus of five lectures and five experiential sessions in Vipassana, Preksha Dhyan and Sahaj Rajayoga of Brahma kumaris in the first academic term from first MBBS to Final MBBS shall ensure first-hand experience of three most prominent evidence-based meditations for health. This teaching and training shall create belief and faith in the ancient yog systems which have become key strategies for health in USA. Dr. Mhaisekar, present VC of MUHS is trying his best to implement this add-on syllabus as a stress buster for the medical students wef June 2018. Recommendations of Dr. Kaundinya Committee have been sent in toto to the MCI after discussion in the Academic Council of MUHS. But the reality is different. MCI is non-functional. Secondly, an add-on syllabus for upgrading and bringing the existing MCI approved syllabus to global level [five lecture and five practical experiential sessions] does not require MCI approval. It could be done at University level only. Honourale VC Dr. Mhaisekar has promised to do it with the support of next Academic council.

Such positive steps give a hope that distant dream of health for all shall become a reality very soon.

Spirituality Religion, and God

The term Spiritual pertains to spirit, soul, atman or Rooh. Different religions call the same entity by different names. The same happens with the belief system about God. Scriptures and also various religions tell us that there is only One God, One and The Only One, The Supreme. But in the same breath Hindus talk about 33 crores of Gods and Goddesses. This is quite confusing and more so to the scientist minds. This confusion is at its best in the present iron era which scriptures call as the era of mass mental confusion **[Bhrusht Mati]**. All the religions believe that God is incorporeal and in the form of bright effulgent light. Only Hindus worship body forms like Ram, Krishna, Shankar and several others. Kufra is a major sin in Holy Quran. It is committed when a man worships anything else other than the One and The Only One Allah. This concept of One avoids all confusion and results in unshakable faith. Both Islam and Hinduism are way of life or art of living as they show a Straight Path, Sirat al mustaqim or Path of Shreyas. Quran tells — The believers shall survive and thrive. But the no-believers shall suffer and perish. BK-Rajayoga calls the Divine guidance for avoiding Devil's path as **Shrimat. The concept of God** should be acceptable to whole of the human race. So obviously Ram, Krishna, Shankar and other body forms could not be the Supreme One and The Only One. Under these dubious circumstances when each one feels that his/her God is good and greater than others, it becomes necessary to know precisely- Who is God? The best person to tell it is God Himself. Holy Quran says – Devil has challenged All Merciful Allah that he shall lure away all of His beloved children into his clutches and to their final doom. Present times and incidences are proving it to the maximum.

God is All Merciful. So He created in-built **anti-devil mechanisms** in Human Beings, a **BMSO- Body Mind Soul Organism**. These programs in BMSO try their best to prevent a man from going into the clutches of Devil. Charak Sanhita, 1000 years ago, described five Body-sheaths surrounding the **core personality or Atman**- Outermost is Annamaya kosh, pranamaya kosh, manamaya kosh, gyan-vigyanmaya kosh and innermost is anandmaya kosh. Modern drugs act only up to Annamaya kosh. This may be one of the reasons for the absence of their effectiveness. Gyan-vigyanmaya kosh is the famous "Inner voice"[Antar-mana] which shouts the loudest when a man is about to commit a bad karma. If karma is repeated often this inner voice goes on become feebler and feebler. Second system consists of a Reward Centre, Punishment centre and Reverberating circuits in the brain. A Good karma activates Reward centre releasing "Feel Good Hormones'. A Bad karma stimulates Punishment centre releasing damaging stress hormones. Both the effects are maintained for a long time because of the Reverberating circuits. The stress hormones eventually give rise to various chronic diseases, pain and suffering **[Bhog].** Holy Quran describes a Godly deterrent. Two angels on each shoulder record each every act that is performed. At the time of reckoning [Kayamat] Merciful Allah becomes a stern judge. He shows a reel of all bad karma. Clever man protests and tells his picture is morphed. Then two angels give their witness. Hinduism has Chitragupta keeping all the records. Man once again protests and tells these witnesses have been purchased by some other sinner. At this point of time, the organ with which sin was committed starts giving witness. Punishment then is given in accordance with the gravity of the sin.

Hinduism **[Garuda purana]** mentions horrible punishments for various types of sins. Bhagavad Gita tells about **Bhog** i.e. pain and sufferings in life which are of four kinds- of body, mind, people and money.

A recent study has shown that the lifespan of an average Indian has been increased by 20 years. But unfortunately, all of these bonus years are spent in sufferings due to **chronic incurable diseases** in which Quality Of Life **[Q.O.L.]** is a victim. Bhagavad Gita calls it as **karma Bhog.** Spiritual wisdom calls this is as an **End stage battle** of the soul. The bad karmic account is shed by suffering. **Other way of shedding the karmic load** is by single pointed remembrance of God.

Indian, Egyptian, and Greek philosophies believe in **Golden age** and **golden race [with Kanchan Kaya]** in which life is heavenly with no knowledge about God and there is an absence of any religion. Holy Quran also tells that a day shall come when all the human beings shall lose faith on God because of the numerous religions and their subsects created by the **selfish people for self gain and exploitation.** All Merciful Allah then give His Message to a chosen few **[Wahi]** who are selfless and fearless for spreading the message to the masses. All different religions shall then vanish and a single religion- that of humanity shall emerge.

BK-Rajayog, God and Soul

Each soul passes through four stages of Yog- karma yog, japa yog, Bhakti yog and Gyan Yog or Rajayoga. Author has undergone the experience of ten different paths before finally realizing that Brahma Kumaris Rajayoga is easy, ultimate and most precise. My japa yog began when my friend advised to chant Om Namo shivaya thousand times in a day for one month when I was passing through a very difficult period in my life. All the measures have failed to solve the problem. Mind was superfast with worries and pressures. So chanting was very rapid, hurried and mechanical. On 21st day the desired miracle happened. Gross injustice that had happened was rectified. I believed at that point of time that God has given me pain and suffering and I used to ask-why me? The knowledge gained from a week of foundation course of BrahmaKumaris made realize that it is my bad karmic account that gave Bhog and not the God. A change happened in my chanting mode after this emancipation of a sort. Chanting became slow. The pause between each word became utilized for visualization and for dwelling in the "Blissful Experience." Each word got repeated with love, belief, faith and total trusting surrender. This was the beginning of loveful, peaceful and blissful Bhakti Yog. **Different kinds of chanting** which include chanting of Gayatri mantra, Omkar meditation, repeatedly uttering the, names of the Lord Krishna or Mahesh or of a **Kalama in Holy Quran**; give quietness of the turbulent judgmental Scientist mind [Antar-mauna-Internal silence]. The powerful and knowledgeful Spiritualist Mind then comes on forefront managing the various mental and physical processes in BMSO-Body Mind Soul Organism or man. Turbulence in mind indicates a Body-conscious state while the peaceful state shows dominance of Spiritualist Mind and it is known as Soul conscious state. **Bhagavad Gita tells that all the pain and sufferings in life arise out of body conscious state of mind.** In soul conscious state an Atman to Atman transpersonal human transactions happen in which two participants are equal-the children of the Supreme Soul or God. If each one believes in this concept and modify his/her behavior, then the dream of **global brotherhood** shall become a reality within a short time.

The preponderance of this mind also denotes soul conscious state. The soul conscious state of mind is indicated by **shavasan** and **Ekagra chitta avastha** [Patanjali Sutra]. Dr. Herbert Benson, an American cardiologist, and the founder of first Institute of Mind and Body Medicine in USA in 1970 coined two terms-Biological Relaxation Response **[B.R.R.] and "The Zone"** for the ancient terms. But **Macaulay-programmed Indian minds** find it difficult to believe and have faith in ancient Indian Shavasan and Ekagra chitta avastha. After all they firmly believe that whatever is Western or British is good and greater than our own.

The enhanced focus of mind in tranquil state **enhances performance.** I know a medical student in Sir J J Hospital who started in ISKCON when H.H. Gaurang Prabhu used to come for his superb sermons. This student who was also chanting the mahamantra- **"Hare Rama Hare Ram, Ram Ram hare hare, hare Krishna hare Krishna, Krishna Krishna hare hare"** apart from his studies created an unbeatable record by winning ten **Gold medals in Final M.B.B.S. examination. Wonderful sermons by H.H. Devamrut, H.H. Gaurang Prabhu then and by H.H. Gaur Gopal Prabhu** and H.H. Shubh Vilas Prabhu now, facilitated my spiritual enlightenment and spiritual evolution.

The reason I went to ISKCON was I felt an **ill defined emptiness** within. Dr. N.N. Wig, Professor emeritus of Psychiatry, P.G.I., Chandigarh, coined the term **"Spiritual Vacuum"** for this emptiness in life in spite of various achievements and happiness in life. Eventually this state leads to weakening of mind and soul and results in the loss of power to differentiate between morally wrong and right **[Vivek-shunyata].** Such person then prefers **Devil's Path** for quick material gains and high achievements. **[High Achiever's syndrome].**

This Divine Grace comes to those whose past karmic account is good at a pre-ordained point of time in one's life. The person continues to overlook the proffered hand of God Himself for Divine help in the absence of Divine Grace. Thus I went a seven days' foundation course in the concepts of Brahma Kumaris organization. This meant a quantum jump in precise understanding of the spiritualism. Fortunately this Free of cost course is available at the BK-Meditation Hut in the divine campus of Sir J J Hospital, Mumbai. I believe and have experienced that this hospital campus is Divine. It came into existence because of the exceptional philanthropy of a generous soul, Sir Jamshetjee Jeejeebhoy who donated his entire life earnings for the divine cause. Soon, within a year, as **pre-ordained Divine Plan** I went to Mount Abu. This was a minor miracle. This is because the Centre in charges have **several sieves for filtering out the souls worth sending to Mount Abu.** BK-organization is a global N.G.O. with consultative status in U.N.O. and it has won 6 international awards for its efforts to bring global peace. It has won the highest state award for De-addiction work in eight districts of Maharashtra for last three consecutive years. Mount Abu open heart trial, initiated by Honorable President Abdul Kalam in year 1998 has given the miracle of reversal of heart disease. **R.E.R.F.** [Rajayoga Education and Research Foundation] and Medical/S.P.A.R. C. wing has a novel **Thought Graph machine** which can demonstrate the result of his meditative practice and transformation of Negative mindset [**Vrutti**] into a positive one. Once convinced, I included BK-Rajayoga in my daily routine. Soon I discovered that this practice is habit forming because of the release of **natural endogenous endorphin** which is not harmful. Eventually my seven incurable diseases vanished because of the

God's pharmacy released during mindfulness. This PMF-Primary Motivational Factor for continuing the practice of Rajayoga later on transformed into a spiritual quest for attaining deity-like status eventually. One has to **"Experience" the cosmic flow** of inspirations coming to us during deep meditative states for believing in them. These divine directions are specific in nature and help to realize our weaknesses and to strengthen our strengths. I now realize why **Swami Vivekananda** said-'Nobody teacheth anybody. Each one teacheth himself [under divine guidance]. Focus and **S.W.O.T-analysis** along with an **Out of Box thinking** happens which gives innovative solutions to the problems of various kinds. **A cosmic Google** forewarns about impending dangers and protects from catastrophes. This is what is known as **sixth sense**, premonition, intuition or gut feeling which motivates to travel for an extra mile to achieve your goals. **Split second decisions** turn out to be very accurate and the best. Malcolm Gladwell discusses this "Blink phenomenon" or **the power of thinking without thinking** in his book. Another peculiar "Experience" is that every day some **positive stroke** happens that goes on strengthening your **belief and faith to an unshakable level.**

It is noteworthy that both Holy Quran and the spiritual concepts became available to the suffering mankind through "Mystical experiences" [**Sakshatkars**]. Incorporeal God gives His Message through a human conduit of highly evolved and enlightened souls known as Messiah or Messengers of God. Neuroscience shows that both Hallucinations [Bhrum] and the mystical experiences occur in the same area of brain. So the most common question from the doctors is why BK-spiritual concepts are not hallucinations? Psychiatrists describe a mental affliction called as **Scientism**. Such mindsets do not believe in anything unless it is proved by science. They do not realize the depth when Sir **Albert Einstein** said- "Science is but an infant." [It never can grasp the vast expanse of divinity in Toto]. Mere glance at the history of medicine shows that the progress in science takes the man from the areas of greater errors to those with lesser errors. But whatever the stage of progress, an area always remains unknown to man. This is the domain of God where miracles happen. Blood lymphocyte was a phlegmatic spectator gathering at the periphery of an inflammatory focus before the year 1960. But when **Burnet [Australia] and Medawar [England]** discovered the subset populations of lymphocytes and their interleukins, suddenly it became a Brigadier orchestrating the intense life and death battle between invading bacteria and defending polymorphs.

In short science could never be able to demonstrate the existence of God and Soul. But they do exist.

BRAHMA KUMARIS SPIRITUAL CONCEPTS AND RAJAYOGA

Incorporeal Supreme Soul **[Param-atma]**, Shiva, chooses a human conduit, Dada Lekhraj, an internationally renowned diamond merchant based in Karachi. He became known as Brahma Baba after the mystical experiences which gave the spiritual knowledge. BK-Rajayoga is a precise spiritual practice done under Divine guidance called as Shrimat which is received through "Muralis" read at specific times in all of the 11500 BK-centers in 140 countries.

The author has a personal experience of last 21 years that any question or doubt gets immediately solved **through Murali read at the BK-centre** on the next day. It feels as if the Supreme Himself is holding our hands and guiding us through the turbulences of modern life. The BK-concepts are very precise, logical and very easy to understand. ISKCON experience showed me that a simple technique of connecting to God becomes a very lengthy, tiresome and complex because of the several fear generating terms and conditions. **Ten types of sins** can happen if chanting is not done in a particular way. Prostration in front of deities in temple has to be in a particular way. Otherwise it is pointed out that your feet are pointing to some Prabhu or other. **This again becomes a sin. If Krishna or God is omnipresent**, in the floor tiles also, then we all are committing the gravest sin of walking over Krishna. Thereupon I asked a question. How we can protect ourselves from this sin? It remains unanswered even today. Equating Krishna with deities like Shiva or Vishnu also became a sin. The question who is Vishnu or Shiva remained unanswered. Another very pertinent question is how Krishna can be the Supreme God when Muslims, Christians and others do not believe in Him as God. All the religions believe that God is effulgent bright white light. Everybody says "God is One and the Only One." Then why there are 33 crores of Gods and Goddesses only in Hinduism? **Who is this dubious King, Indra?** Why he always lies in the shadow of fear of losing his throne whenever one does intense sadhana? How and why does he have a license to maintain a harem of beautiful Apsaras? Who has authorized him to go on sending beautiful damsels for breaking the purity of a sadhak? The questions in Bhakti were unending. **H.H. Gaurang Prabhu, H.H. Gaur Gopal Prabhu and H.H. Shubh Vilas Prabhu**, all of them have brilliant minds and they know Bhagavad Gita and Shrimad Bhagavatam by heart including the Shlokas in Sanskrit. Their lectures created an inferiority complex and information **highway stress**. I pessimistically started believing that emancipation for me is not going to happen in this birth. It was a sad and wrong conclusion. Thus Bhakti yog made me a storehouse of fears, trepidation, low self-esteem, superstitions and blind faith.

BK-concepts as told by God Himself removed all the doubts. **Who is God?** This is a common question in questing mind. I believe the correct answer could be given by God Himself. All others shall only be a concept. Anybody else shall give his own misinformation about the real entity. So BK-concepts obtained from incorporeal Supreme Soul through mystical experiences to an evolved soul became gospel truth for me. I now wonder if **Supreme Godhead in ISKCON** really means Supreme Soul.

BK-concepts are easy, precise and removed many of my fears-
1] Yog or meditation means connecting two infinitely small Points – God and the soul for drawing the powers and inspiration from **Supreme Father of all the souls**, Supreme Teacher and Supreme Sadgatidata.

2] Soul- I am not this body. But I am a soul, a conscient, metaphysical extremely tiny point situated in the centre of the forehead in between the eyebrows. This site is also known as: "Third eye", Spiritual eye or Agya energy chakra. Western scientists call the **pineal gland** situated in the same axis as **God's spot** as soul is believed to be present there.

3] God – is also tiny, metaphysical, conscient point of light. But He is ocean of power, Knowledge and purity. He is timeless, ageless, limitless, birth -less and death-less.

4] We human beings are the 33 crores of Deities who descend to the present deteriorated level because of contamination of consciousness by Vasana [desires], Vikalpa [negative thoughts], Vikara [negative emotions] and Vikshepa [distorted perception due to bad experiences in the past]. Maya, Ravana or Devil is this **negativity of mind.** The goal of **spiritual effort [Purusharth]** is for regaining the deity status once again. Thus we are not human beings who are undergoing spiritual experience but in reality we are the spiritual beings who are undergoing human experience in accordance with our karma of last birth. **Past Life Regression Hypnosis** [P.L.R.H.] therapy in psychiatry proves that a soul passes through eternal cycles of life and death.

5] Time cycle- Total duration of one time cycle [Kaal chakra] is only five thousand years. It is equally divided into 4 eras- Golden age, Silver, Copper and Iron Age. Last couple of hundred years forms an era of confluence [Sangam Yug]. This is the era for total spiritual effort for achieving **Karmateet avastha** [Total soul conscious state] and for regaining deity status. The time cycle is repeating eternally from an unknown beginning. So a fossil which is thirty thousand years old in age should not be a surprise.

6] Soul passing through 84 thousand yonis or animal species is a myth. A human being always takes birth as human being only. There are only 84 births. **This was a**

great relief to me. I used to worry that if I become a tiger or lion or a shark in next birth because of my fish and meat eating saraswat habit, then how I could switch over to vegetarian diet for once again getting a human birth?

7] Bad Karmic account of previous births results in pain, Suffering, diseases, premature deaths, failures and poverty [**Bhog**]. There are two ways of shedding or burning out this karmic load- One is by suffering and secondly by remembrance of Supreme Soul with single pointed focus , i.e. by volcanic meditation. I now firmly believe that my relief from cervical spondylitits, chronic cough, unstable angina, Thyrotoxicosis, severe back pain due to spondyolisthesis and complete healing of my tendo-achilles tear happened because my karmic account got burnt by fire of meditation [**Yogagni**].

8] **God never gives pains and sufferings.** He gives only happiness and peace in life and gives divine guidance for spiritual effort.

Science Behind God, Soul and Health

God is an enigma even today when scientific developments are so much advanced. An atheist totally disbelieves in the existence of God. Agnostic holds a belief that nothing is known or likely to be known of the existence of God or of anything beyond material phenomena. Scientism is a mindset that is ready to believe in the existence of God if proved by science. On the other hand millions in the whole word believe that God exists and He is always Merciful and helping. So the concepts may differ according to the perception, belief [Bhav] and Faith [shruddha] of a person.. Milestones in the history of religions and spiritualism reveal that whole of the spiritual knowledge has been a conglomerate of divine "Experiences" and "Mystical experiences" of highly evolved and enlightened souls. World calls them Mesiha or Messengers of God. The Message of God is always delivered through these Messengers like Mohamad Paigamber, Jesus Christ, Mahaveer, Gautam Buddha, Zorastrua and others. Brahma Kumaris Rajayog concepts are from mystical experience to a human conduit, Brahma Baba given by incorporeal God. Doctors refuse to believe in such mystical experiences because both hallicinations [Bhrum] and Mystical experiences [Sakshatkars] occur in the same area of cerebral cortex. So it has been my experience that they dismiss BK-Rajayoga as myth, hallucination, superstition or blind faith. They refuse to believe in the "Experiential evidences of miracles" by millions of people. Ancient Ayurveda and Unani derive conclusions based on Experiential evidence" which does not require costly equipments and instruments for proof of the cure. Problem again is that modern mainstream medicine stubbornly refuses to publish anything that is not proved by scientific experiments. This rigidity for publishing becomes a greater hurdle for publishing cures by herbs. Modern medicine demands to know active ingradient. A herb contains more than 40 different components. Some of which may be healing. Others or all may not be having curing property at all. But a synergistic action may contribute to cure. Thus to prove that a herb ingradient is curing may require lifetime research. Ingenuous China bypassed this obstacle by creating a Database, Qi Long Database compiling all the unpublished research on Tai Chi, chinese form of meditation and cure by herbs. Thus China has now captured world market in the field of Complementary Alternative Medicine (CAM). There is an urgent need to form an Indian database of this kind for yoga research. I have personally experienced hurdles in publication of material related to Brahma kumaris Rajayog.

The health scenario today is full of mass confusion which is said to be the predominant feature of iron age [Kali-yug] in scriptures. There are multiple therapies, approaches and techniques. So a wide arena for exploitation of the gullibles becomes open to the quacks with their unsubstantiated claims of "Miracle cures". In spiritualism also there are multiple Paths, Gurus, Sadgurus and self proclaimed Gods. Scriptures of all religions tell "There is Only One God, The One and The Only One, the Supreme." But Hindus believe in 33 crores of different Gods and Godesses. Holy Quran calls this act as Kufra meaning gravest sin of worshiping anything else other than The One and the Only One. All the religions prescribe that man should follow a Straight Path, Sirat al mustaqim or Path of Shreyas. But in actual life follow Devil's Path. Devil first makes a man totally confused [Bhrusht Mati] and then gradually leads to final destruction by diseases in pain and suffering. N.C.D.s- Non-infectious Chronic Diseases like Diabetes, Depression and cancer provide the proof. AIDS is the result of Bad karma. HIV comes much later in the picture. The root cause is mind or Dil which is not under control and goes on demanding more and more and also instant gratification of sensual and sexual pleasure and craving for materialistic gains. This may be labeled as "High achiever syndrome."

I believe that BK-Concepts about God and soul are gospel truths because they have been told to humanity through mystical experiences. But for the scientists and spiritualists of world today, God remains as an unsolved riddle as they do not as yet know what is meant by consciousness [Chaitanyamaya Shakti]. BK-Rajayoga tells that consciousness means energy having awareness. One thousand years old Charak Sanhita is the first treatise on Whole Person Medicine and Health

Promotion. It describes 15 types of personalities [Prakruti] depending on consciousness. Sheldon's classification in contrast describes only Three Morphotypes- Body types- Ecto, Meso and endomorph and their correlation to diseases.

Advance in the field of Artificial Intelligence [AI] has brought miraculous working intelligence in Robots. But even today the Emotional Intelligence [E.Q.] could not be incorporated in the Robotics. This is because only consciousness grants the ability of a doer, feeler and creator of emotions to the man.

A confused vicious mind cannot visualize and experience God and divine powers and qualities. So it demands scientific proof for God's existence. It is like asking for a DNA report from our parents for proving their parentage. All Merciful God, it seems is now ready to provide scientific proof also.

Alchemy of God consists of a group of young BK-scientists from S.P.A.R.C.[Spiritual Advancement Research Centre] Wing of Brahma Kumaris. They proposed a novel CQSE [Consciousness Quantum Spiritual Energy] for soul, Supreme Conscious Unified G Force [gravity and levity] of Universe for God and for Universe [Brahmand] using principles of sacred or divine geometry. This novel concept was presented in world congress of scientists working on artificial intelligence in 2016 and in 2017 in USA. Scientist world now has a storm.

Ancient scripture Shrimad Bhagavatam describes that soul is very tiny. When you cut a tip of hair ten thousand times then each of the segments may represent the size of the soul. Hardcore mindsets afflicted with scientism believe that they shall be able to believe in the existence of God and soul when the research on Neutrino in NOL- Neutrino Observatory Laboratory in Bengaluru completes its research in 2050. This is height of sheer mindless optimism because spiritual wisdom tells that no one can guarantee the next moment of your life. Neutrino is the tiniest known inert particle which has the highest speed may be like that of mind, the third component of a soul.

CQSE CONCEPT OF ALCHEMY OF GOD

CQSE- Consciousness Quantum Spiritual Energy or soul is a sacred geometrical structure. Its size is beyond even Planck scale of measurement. It is very subtle quantum gravity whose basic frequency acts on human brain by creating vibrations in Aether [Quantum Vacuum Energy medium]. Electromagnetic photons from this energy field act on microtubules of neurons through a sacred geometrical energy field [Aura or Aether]. There are 16 Aether Energy Points in CQSE which forms the basis of life force energy [Prana]. This energy passes to various organs and cells of the body through seven main and 6 minor energy chakras. Seven main energy chakras from top to bottom are Sahasara, Agya, Vishuddhi, Anahat, Manipura, Swadhishthan and the lowest one called Muladhar chakra. Scriptures tell that a soul leaves the body at the time of death from Sahasara chakra if the man pursued a straight path throughout his life. A satanic life makes the soul leave the body through Muladhar chakra. Agya chakra is also known as the Third Eye or Spiritual eye [Divya chakshu]. It distributes energy to whole of the nervous system and Pituitary gland and as such is the controller of all the physical and biochemical processes in the body. Vishuddhi chakra provides energy to neck structures and Thyroid and parathyroid glands. Anahat is for chest organs- heart and lungs. Manipura is for Gastro-intestinal tract. Swadhishthan is the energy provider for genito-urinary system. Muladhar is responsible for energy to genital glands.

CQSE or soul is like a pentagonal star with angles of 18, 36, 72, and 108 degrees. It has 16 Aether energy points. Operating system of CQSE is in the form of mind, intellect and traits or impressions. They lie in the points number one to three. Remaining 13 points include five elements of nature [Prakruti] namely air, fire, water, Aether and sky] followed by values and divine qualities. All of these 16 energy points are connected to energy chakras in subtle body [Sukshma sharir]. Mind, intellect and traits are the three different manifestations of consciousness in the soul [CQSE]. Mind is a virtual screen on which thoughts and emotions or desires are formed as transient waves. Thought signals generated by mind are given to intellect for analyzing right or wrong in accordance with Divine Universal or cosmic laws which are applicable to all the human beings. The decision by intellect gives signal for action [Karma]. Mind acts both as the transmitter and receiver of the signals. The decision by intellect produces a basic vibration frequency which is decoded by a particular group of neurons in Hypothalamus. This in turn triggers neurons in Pituitary and Thalamus which functions as relay station for passing on the vibration to specific neurons in brain capable of producing desired action [Karma] or physical activity. The vibration impulse is passed to the target organs or structures through the nerves and energy chakras. The karma results in a feeling or emotion which is registered by mind. Thus mind acts both as a transmitter and the receiver; or the doer, the observer and also he feeler of emotions.

Repeated desires [vasana], negative thoughts [vikalpa] and negative emotions [vikara] result in karma under propitious circumstances. Emotion means a thought which has a power to initiate action or karma. At first, the internal warning system, inner voice shouts the loudest and tells not to commit an unethical act. But as the karma gets repeated, this warning system becomes feebler and feebler and a habit is formed. Spiritual wisdom tells that a habit is difficult to cure. This is because you remove H, abit remains. You remove A. Bit remains. You remove B. It remains. Then what is the solution? Remove I or ego. This shall allow T or transformation to occur. The power to remove I or ego comes from Meditation. Unchecked habit eventually results in formation of the nature [Vrutti] which decides the perception, attitude and behavioral pattern of a person. This nature is carried to the next birth by the soul [CQSE] as traits [sanskars] or a spiritual genome. It is not a small wonder that some children are satanik or devilish right from birth.

Child prodigies, reincarnation and Out of Body experiences [O.B.E. or N.D.E. Near Death Experience] and Past Life Regression hypnosis/Therapy [P.L.R.T.] prove that soul exists and traits are transferred to the next birth.

SECRETS OF ENERGY OF UNIVERSE

Alchemy of God and a novel book by **David Wilcock** – entitled "The Source Field Investigations-The hidden science and lost civilizations behind the 2012 prophecies" give a detail scientific description of an unknown benevolent inexhaustible Energy which is running the Universe precisely and flawlessly for eternal number of years.

WHO IS GOD?

Alchemy of God tells that God is Supreme Consciousness Unified G Force [gravity and levity both are present] of Universe and it occurs in the Tenth Dimension of Universe. A common man like me knows that even a fourth dimension of reality may exist. But tenth dimension is simply outrageous. The force has a high Quantum Vacuum Energy commonly known as Aether. It consists of 10 raised to 21 GeV of energy and has an infinite silence field of pure consciousness. The purity of consciousness is of utmost importance in spiritual efforts [Purusharth] because of this reason. The Supreme consciousness manifests in the entire universe with the help of super strings [String Theory] in tenth dimension and creates 16 types of Aether energies. The Universal original energy that runs the entire universe functions on love, peace, purity, bliss, power and knowledge. So it is not a wonder that all of these divine qualities form the inherent qualities of CQSE or soul.

WHAT IS AETHER ELEMENT OR THE CONSCIOUS ZERO POINT OF ENERGY?

Nature [Prakruti] consists of five elements- earth, water, fire, air and sky. Aether is the sixth element [Brahma Tatva] of the cosmic world having consciousness. This conscious form of energy spins [Torsion waves] and gives rise to the five elements of nature. Aether is also known as Life-force energy [Prana]. Aether energy exists at a very subtle value of 10 raised to minus 35. But its entire infinite energy comes from torsion waves.

WHAT IS UNIVERSE [BRAHMAND]?

Universe is a creation of the Supreme Creator, God or Supreme Conscious Unified Field. Various activities in Universe get manifested through certain fundamental patterns of energy, frequency and vibrations. There are three fundamental energy components which act synergistically to manifest everything in Universe [Theory of Everything TOE] :-

1]   Vector tensegrity- geometric patterns and structures.

2]   Torus flow process- Primary form of energy in motion as a whirl pool.

3]   Field patterning- Wave interaction of vector, tensegrity and torus flow dynamics.

A unique geometric structure of five elements exists in each of the three components with Fibonacci numbers and Golden ratio

These two are the basic requirement for creation of matter as well as different forces of nature [Prakruti].

All of the above mentioned secrets of Universe may be within the grasp of a scientist. But in medical world, all of this becomes an illegible jargon. This is the proof that a most brilliant human intellect may know as little as a drop in the ocean of knowledge. It is a miracle that the energy running the entire Universe eternally and flawlessly is inexhaustible. Scientists have not discovered such kind of fuel. Another miracle is that a tiny seed has all the potential to grow into a huge Bunyan tree or a mango tree. All of this indicates the presence of a Supreme Power with Supreme Intelligence having a Supreme creativity of a Supreme Creator. Man is a BMSO- Body Mind Soul Organism. This superb machine is controlled by tiny Powerful Points- God, Soul, Energy chakras, cerebral genes [Allen's Brain map], somatic genes and receptors. More than 200 oncogenes exist in the body. Each one of them is capable of giving a specific form of cancer. It is small wonder that most of us do not develop cancer even though we are functioning in an atmosphere full of carcinogens. This miracle could be explained on the basis of karma theory in Bhagavad Gita. Minor degree of Vikarma [Bad act] may give minor health problems. Major sins may result is chronic incurable diseases with pain and suffering till death.

Super Quantum Gravity [SQG] energy field of God [Supreme Universal Conscious energy] or Energy aura is pentagonal in shape and has 32 energy points in it. These Points are the source of various forms of infinite or unlimited energies. Three sub-energy levels are used for Creation and Governance, for operations, maintenance or preservation and finally for the destruction of the effete and evil. This is famous Trinity of Brahma, Vishnu and Mahesh. Most amazing feature is that this Unified field has its own memory and consciousness. TOE –Theory of Everything tells that specific vibration- states give rise to specific kinds of particles and corresponding matter as well as different forms of energy in this material world. This energy field exists at the seventh energy level of Universe. This may explain why there are seven levels of Samadhi or spiritual evolution. A man could perform super human acts [Siddhis] like clairvoyance, levitation, walking on fire or water or astral travel at higher levels of spiritual evolution. This intelligent energy field knows the past, present and future in very precise terms.[Trikaldarshi]. This Energy field is beyond the set rules of time, space and matter. It has a power to change time and space of the Universe. It can create or destroy multiple universes like ours very easily and at any moment.

Thirty two Energy points have a specific divine quality or power.eg.- Love, Peace, bliss, power of rejuvenating or destroying, liberation from death, knowledge of the past, present and future, bestowing happiness, removing sorrows, bestowing of Divine intellect and others.

David Wilcock in his book describes a benevolent, mutagenic and healing all pervasive energy of the Universe which is termed as Source Field. We shall know about the various miracles brought about by the Egyptian pyramids through this Source Field.

POWER YOGA BY ALCHEMY OF GOD

BK-concepts define meditation as establishing a CONNECTION between the soul with Supreme –Soul [Param-atma] for drawing the rays and vibrations of power and peace and purity from the supreme powerhouse. This confers three astounding powers to the soul- **Self-determination, Self-dedication** and **self-discipline** which are required for success in any task and in any life situation. These three in turn give tremendous self-esteem which does not allow a person to compromise on values and ethics. Power yoga of Alchemy of God involves a complex process of visualization in which 132 Points of Power in Supreme Consciousness are connected with corresponding points of energy with specific colors in CQSE-Consciousness Quantum Spiritual Energy. I experimented with this technique and found it very lengthy and tedious as compared to God given BK-Rajayoga. A common man like me cannot fathom the deep science guaranteeing very powerful experience and quick empowerment by the practice of Power Yoga.

Source Field, Edgar Cyace Readings, Golden Age and Pyramid Healing Power

David Wilcock, in his amazing book "Source Field Investigations, The Hidden Science and Lost civilizations Behind The 2012 prophecies" describes an Universal , all pervasive, benevolent, mutagenic and healing energy of unknown nature which has been termed as Source Field. Author believes that this Source Field is same as Aether described in previous chapter by Alchemy Of God. Recently, in 2014, scientists have discovered an unknown form of protective energy that is surrounding the earth like a sheath. They also discovered a cosmic fusillade of lethal electrons which have a capacity to make the earth disappear in smoke in fraction of a second. The shield provided by the unknown energy is protecting us.

EDGAR CAYCE READINGS- [JUNE 30-1932]
Edgar Cayce was a noteworthy psychic reader in early twentieth century. Cayce's readings came from what he spoke when he was put in a hypnotic stance. These readings are surprisingly similar to what has been known as **Vedantic principles** in Bhagavad Gita, Mahabharat and in Hindu scriptures.

Cayce told that we all have a soul, [called as Atman in Bhagavad Gita] which constantly keeps a watch over us while also enjoying life's experiences, thoughts and emotions. Any one of us could reach this subtle aspect of our existence or Being [sukshma sharir] and can get the ability to understand the greater plan and purpose of our lives which has been chosen before we came here on planet earth. [**Pre-ordained Divine Plan** decided by the karma in previous birth]. Process of enlightenment could save us a great deal of needless pain and suffering in this life. But when we resist this reality and purpose we encounter only more and more sufferings and difficulties in our lives that we label as **bad luck**. All of this happens in accordance with eternal spiritual laws of which law of karma is one. Whatever we measure out to others will be measured back to us. Ignorance of spiritual laws does not grant exemption. If we violate some one's free will, then the measure shall be so great that sometimes we may require another life time to balance it out by enduring similar hardships. Cayce further tells that we can eliminate the entire cycle of karma by practicing true forgiveness and acceptance of our faults, both of ourselves and of others. Cayce also told about the disturbances of nature today like wars, terrorism, corruption in government, natural disasters, earthquakes and floods. As you sow, so you reap.

Cayce's Readings spoke of God as Universal Loving Intelligence that does not discriminate against anyone. But we do and therefore there are more wars and more bloodshed on the basis of racial and religious differences. Lord is One and The Only One. We fight believing that our God is greater and The Only One.

Tsunamis of the physical world are because of tsunamis of violence in human consciousness.

Cayce told about the catastrophes happening at the end of Kali Yug that was described in Hindu scriptures like Bhagavad Gita and Mahabharata. Kali Yug is an era of mass corruption and moral decline. Sinful monarchs addicted to false speech shall govern their subjects on the principles that are false. The merchants shall be full of guile. They shall sell large quantities of merchandise with false weights and measures. Those who are virtuous shall not prosper. The sinful shall prosper exceedingly. Virtues shall lose the strength while sins shall become very powerful. Girls aged 7 or 8 years shall conceive. Women shall deceive the best husbands. Lives of men shall become very short. Brahmins shall abstain from prayers and meditation. This shall be final stage in kali yug. Surprisingly newspapers are confirming that all of this is happening today after so many years.

At the end of kali Yug seven blazing Suns shall appear and shall give a devastating fire, called **Samvartaka**. This fire shall destroy all things in a moment. But surprisingly the story after this cataclysm continues. That means everyone is still alive right after everything is allegedly destroyed by incredible fire. A savior figure, **Kalki** with super natural powers shall appear who shall defeat the bad guys and shall transforms this planet. Kalki shall be able to manifest vehicles, weapons and warriors just by thinking about them. He shall be the person who shall possess great intelligence and great energy. The creation shall begin anew and **Krita or Golden Age** shall arrive.

Hindu scriptures tell that Golden Age shall start to restore the balance of nature and cosmos creating prosperity, abundance, health and peace. Sin shall be rooted out. Brahmins will become good, honest and devoted to ascetic austerities. They shall become **Muni or Silent Meditators.** Men shall begin to honor and practice truth. The men who are thus changed shall give birth to a race that shall follow the laws of Golden Age. It is possible that Brahma Kumars who meditate for deep silence and prove the power of silence through manasa seva for bringing in the global peace are these silent meditators or Munis. Purity is the law in Golden Age. Brahma Kumaris organization stresses that a practitioner of BK-Rajayoga should have utmost level of purity in his karma and in his mind. This is the deity-like status of the people in Golden Age.

Hindu scriptures give us a precise Time Window for when the Golden Age will arrive. The advent of Golden Age is associated with a rare configuration of planets. When the Sun, the Moon, the lunar asterism Tishya and Jupiter are in one mansion the Krita or Satya Yug shall return. Seven blazing Suns and the fire appear to symbolize sudden spiritual awakening that happens throughout the humanity. Edward Cayce says that they may also symbolize seven energy chakras in the human body and their fire. BK-concepts call this as the fire of Yog, Yogagni or Volcanic Meditation.

An Egyptian document called **Asclepius's lament** also describes nearly same thing which has been described in Hindu scriptures." When all will be disordered and unholy, then the God, The Creator of all things will call back to the Right path [Sirat al mustaqim in Holy Quran] those who have gone astray. He will cleanse the world of evil washing it away with floods, burning it out with fiercest of fire and expelling with wars and pestilence. Thus He will bring His world to its former aspect. Cosmos will once more be deemed worthy of worship and wondering reverence. Holy Quran also tells us, "that a day shall come when mankind shall lose faith in God and the religion. This is because of the several sub sects of religion created by evil people for selfish gains. At that point of time **All Merciful Allah** shall select a chosen few who shall be fearless and selfless to spread His Message to the mankind, the Vahis, Messiah or Messengers. Believers of the Message shall survive and prosper. The non-believers shall suffer and perish."

We notice today that the prophecy of floods, famine, fires, wars and pestilence has already come true. The prophecy points out to a world in which Gods are no longer on earth meaning Dwaper Yug and Kali-Yug.

Lastly all mythological legends in Eskimos, Romans, Greeks, American Indians, Japanese, Chinese Hindus and Persian speak of final deluge **[Pralaya]** and the Golden race emerging from the deluge. Different cultures all around the world end up with the same exact information.

Mayan race is of aborigines is quite primitive. But surprisingly it predicted exactly the major world events till 2012. Mayan calendar predicted the end of this world in the year 2012 which did not happen. The theory of cosmic consciousness or **Universal Mind** explains why there is similarity in the concepts of different philosophies. This also explains the phenomenon of **Mass Mind Intention** for peace in the world by several people shall actually translate into global peace and also the phenomenon of **Remote Sensing** in which the person may see certain events in future. The phenomenon of simultaneous discoveries by two individuals who are residing miles apart from each other is also explained by the concept of Universal Mind. For example - Medawar in England and burnet in Australia simultaneously discovered the concept of subset populations of lymphocytes. This was a great stride in the field of Immunology, the science of vaccines which is protective and auto-immune disorders which shows that antibodies may destroy self-antigens or own tissues. Thus immune system of the body is a double edged weapon. On one side it offers protection against infectious agents and cancer and on the hand it may be lethal to body's own tissues.

PYRAMIDOLOGY

Taylor in 1840 began a 30 years research project about the measurements of the pyramids and their correlation to miraculous healing, preserving, and rejuvenating unknown energy existing in and around the pyramids. The pyramids are located in the exact centre of the earth's land mass- the true **axis mundi**. The likelihood of finding this perfect location by accident is one in three million. This speaks volumes about the extraordinary brilliance of our ancestors. Another miraculous coincidence is that if you calculate average height of the land above sea level with Miami as the lowest and Himalayas as the highest point, you come out with **5449 inches** which is the exact height of the Great pyramid. Gleaming white tiles of extra-ordinarily polished surface cover the pyramid. Even the tiles on NASA space shuttle do not fit so accurately and so closely. The tiles were inscribed with mysterious unintelligible characters, enough to fill ten thousand pages. Pyramid had three different chambers. King's chamber is in red granite and the coffin is of chocolate brown color. The coffin was carved by tubular drills that could cut through granite five hundred times faster than any technology we have today. Work on pyramid began in June 1932, the year in which **Edgar Cayce Readings** began. This is another remarkable coincidence. Colonel Vyse, who re-built the pyramid after a great earthquake, published exact and detail measurements of the Great Pyramid in Egypt that was built in the year 1840. The pyramid inch is slightly longer than the regular inch by mere half of the width of human hair or by 1.00106 **British inches**.

Dr. Alexander Golod began building massive pyramids in Russia in 1990. The pyramid technology is indeed far more advanced than we ever realized. Our science has not yet progressed to the point that we could identify and understand such a high technology.

Bovis in 1970 found out that the garbage can in the King's chamber contained corpses of cats and other small animals. Strangely they did not smell bad but appeared to have perfectly dried out. Bovis then built a thirty inch tall wooden model of the Great pyramid in his home in France. Vegetables, fruits and meat got preserved in pyramid wonderfully. Karel Drbal, radio engineer in Prague repeated Bovis's experiment in 1950 and found that several different animals could be preserved nicely. In 1959, he also discovered that dull razor blades would be sharpened if he placed them in pyramid shaped structure of card board with exact dimensions. He was awarded Czechoslovakian **patent number** 91304 for the Cheops Pyramid razor blade sharpener. In 2001, Dr. Volodymyr Krashnoholovets did electron microscopy and found that pyramid power was able to transform the molecular structure along the cutting edge of a sharpened razor blade. However, an East-West alignment had a clear cut dulling effect on the blade transforming the straight surface of the blade into lumpy bumpy curves on a microscopic level. This is obviously not supposed to happen in conventional and modern science.

Lyall Watson , the author of Super Nature, repeated Bovis's original experiments with eggs, meat and dead mice. He found that the pyramid preserved them very well. The brewers of Czechoslovakian beer tried to change the shape from round to angular containers. But found that the change resulted in deterioration of the quality of beer even though the method of processing remained same. A German research showed that the mice with identical wounds heal more quickly if they were kept in spherical cages. Architects in Canada report a sudden improvement in schizophrenic patients living in trapezoidal hospital wards. All of these findings seem to violate our cherished law of physics.

Our ancient ancestors were so confident about Pyramid Technology that they built pyramids throughout Egypt, South America, Bosnia, Italy, Greece, Slovania, Russia and China. The Bosnian Pyramid of Sun is over twice the size of the Great Pyramid.

Dr. Alexander Golod, in 1990, began building large pyramids within Russia and Ukraine and by 2010 more than fifty pyramids were built. These pyramids had the internal frame work of PVC pipes covered with fibre glass. They were all built to fit the Golden section- the so-called phi ratio of 1 to 1.618. Largest pyramid is 144 feet [44 meters]. Golod also found that any metal in pyramidal structure decreases the pyramid power.

David Wilcock mentions that Pyramid Technology appears to concentrate the Universal intelligent continuing cosmic consciousness called as Source Field for biological, psychological and spiritual healing. Our thoughts have the power to produce measurable affect on this Source Field or Cosmic consciousnees to alter Nature [prakruti], atmosphere and computers. **Our collective minds and the thoughts** seem to create an energy that affects the behaviour of others. Hypnosis, **telekinesis and telepathy** could be cited as examples. BK-concepts tell about a novel Manasa Seva technique by which one can send thought vibrations of peace and happiness to the souls in the whole world. Sadhak or practitioner auto-suggests and visualizes that he is receiving rays and vibrations of peace and happiness from the Supreme soul and sending them to the whole world. Divine Muralis by Supreme soul Shiva tell us that an empowered soul could even transform the satanic traits of others and of Nature into divine traits by this technique.

PYRAMID TECHNOLOGY COULD SAVE THE WORLD

A plethora of research papers on healing, preserving and rejuvenation by using Pyramid technology, inspite of following strictest scientific protocol, were **refused for publication**. The reason was the pressures from million dollars healthcare industry and Energy industry. Pyramid technology would have ruined these profit making industries.

1] A study from Ivanovskii R & D Institute of Virology under Russian Academy of Medical Sciences-

Dr. Klimenko and Dr. Nosik were studying a new anti-viral drug- Venoglobin. A diluted form of drug was stored in pyramid for a few days. It became three times more potent than the original form of drug. Strangely the drug retained its effectiveness even in ultra weak concentrations and showed 300 times more pronounced potency. There is similarity of this situation with principle on which Homeopathy works. Higher dilutions are most effective.It is possible that all pervasive cosmic healing energy becomes concentrated in a powerfully healing laser beam in deep meditative state. Repair, rejuvenation and recharging of depleted life force energy may happen in this fashion. Experiential evidence of the BK-practitioners need to be substantiated by scientific experiments and research.

2] A study Russian R and D Institute of Gynaecology and Pediatrics-

Professor Antonov discovered magical healing powers of pyramid treated distilled water. Some premature babies were given only a few days to live. They were administered a placebo sample of pyramid treated 1ml of 40 % glucose solution. All of these babies recovered completely. One ml of distilled injectible water was used instead of glucose. Same miraculous results were obtained.

3] Dr. Egorova, Russian Academy of Medical sciences, injected two groups of mice with S.typhimurium, a deadly pathogen for mice. One set of mice were kept in pyramid. Magically sixty percent of mice in Pyramid survived.

4] Dr. Egorova gave a nasty carcinogen to group of mice fed with pyramid water. The control group received the same carcinogen but received only ordinary water. Mice drinking pyramid water showed significantly less incidence of tumours.

No side effects were observed in any pyramid experiment.

5] Bogdanov and asociates found that the rabbits and white rats became two hundred percent stronger in endurance if kept in pyramids. This amazing effect could be used for enhancing performance of the atheltes and sports persons. **Dangerous and illegal use of steroids could be avoided**.

6] In Russia, one pair of pyramid shaped mountains exist named as **Brat** or Brother and **Seska** or sister. People on these hills remain healthy, happy and harmonious. Academy of Sciences confirmed that pyramid energy could reduce criminal behaviour, increase love, peace, happiness and health. The scientists set pyramids in a jail housing nearly 5000 prisoners. In few months, most crimes disappeared.

PYRAMID EFFECT ON ECOLOGY

A region in Russia was facing the problem of contamination of drinking water with strontium and other heavy metals. Dr. Golod's pyramids provided the solution. A series of pyramids were built over the area and within few days they were pumping clear drinking water free of impurities.

Russian National Academy of Sciences discovered a clear protection against catastrophic earth changes like famines, floods, hurricane, earthquakes, volcanos and tsunamis in a radius of 500 miles around a pyramid But all of this quickly got labelled as **pseudoscience** under various kinds of pressures.

It was also found that the buildings in the radius of 500 miles around pyramid were 5000 times less likely to be struck by lightening. The volcanic eruption were five times less than in other regions.

Pyramid energy actively deflects storms and severe weather from the area around a pyramid.

The **Ozone hole** sitting over Sligar lake disappeared when a twenty two meter Pyramid was built in the area. In the area of ozone hole healed, transformed and renewed. Soon the fields became covered with flowers. Surprisingly some extinct plants species re-appeared. DNA for these plants probably came from the healing cosmic energy itself.

Golod built a series of pyramids on oil wells. The oil under pyramids became 30% thinner and much cleaner. Pyramid processed seeds gave 20 to 100% increase in crop production.

Golod conducted studies of air above and around the pyramids with a Russian instrument called as "**Military Locator**" similar to radar. He detected a circle of an unknown energy around the pyramid which was 300 kilometers wide. The energy was so abundant that you would need every single energy plant in Russia to run for twenty four hours to produce this gigantic amount of energy.

Pyramid power can preserve wine, meat, fish, eggs, fruits, flowers, vegetables and milk for very long periods and that too while retaining their natural flavour and fragrance.

Charak Sanhita, Power of Thoughts, Genesis of Habits, Addiction and Nature and Global Consciousness

Our thoughts form the seeds of our karma and destiny.

~ *Bhagavad Gita*

Science has progressed dramatically. But the term Consciousness[chetana] in ancient Indian scriptures remains an enigma even to the top most scientists in the field of Artificial Intelligence [AI]. Working Intelligence [WI] of robots has improved magically. But the best efforts of the scientists have not been able to endow their robots by Emotional Intelligence [E.Q. Emotional Quotient]. Peace, bliss, happiness, purity and love even today are the unique endowments of a human being, a BMSO- Body Mind Soul Organism. This is because emotions and desires [Vasana, Vikara and Vikshepa] are the type of thoughts that result in karma or action are created by consciousness. Even the plants are a living entity because they have consciousness. A daily dose of loving words to plants results in hastening their growth.

Consciousness or chetana is an unknown form of energy which also has awareness, a unique feature of consciousness. The energyis known as Prana or Life force energy.

TYPES OF CONSCIOUSNESS

1] Soul Consciousness- Dr. Deepak Chopra calls it as microcosm, a limited form of consciousness bounded by limitations of the physical world. It is also known as Suksma sharir.

2] Body consciousness- is related to the physical world and to the material body-sthool sharir.

Charak Sanhita tells about five body sheaths which surrounds the soul or Atman- from outside to inside they are called as Annamaya kosh, Pranamaya kosh, manamaya kosh, Gyan-vigyan maya kosh and Anandmaya kosh. All the modern drugs including those used for mental diseases act only upto superficial most Annamaya kosh. This may be one of the reasons for rise in chronic incurable diseases. Pranayam removes the impurities in Pranamaya kosh. Meditation is the only cure of diseases of mind or manamaya kosh. Gyan-vigyanmaya kosh is the famous "Inner voice" that shouts the loudest when a man is about to commit a karma which is not in accordance with the eternal universal laws of cosmos governing the whole world and all the human beings. Ignorance of these laws is not a protection against their dreadful consequences.

Consciousness in the soul or Atman manifests in three forms- **Mind, Intellect/Wisdom and Traits.**

3] Supra conscious state- This is extra-terrestrial transcendental "experience" or Anubhuti which a soul develops in deep meditative states.

4] Supreme consciousness or God- This consciousness is the Supreme Creator, Governor, Operator, controller and Destroyer of effete, useless and evil in the world. BK concepts tell that this Universal cosmic and benevolent energy that governs, and Operates the cosmic events and Destroys the effete or evil is in the form of a conscient point of light. This tiny Governing Operating and Destroying Point is ocean of power, peace, happiness, knowledge and He is the Supreme Father, Supreme Teacher and Supreme Sadgatidata or emancipator of all the souls in this whole world. Sadagati means   final emancipation from pain and sufferings or a Divine euthanasia.

MIND

Mind, the third component of the soul, has been defined as a virtual screen formed by conscious energy of the soul or Atman on which thoughts, emotions and desires arise as transient images.

Roger Sperry in 1970 gave his famous concept of one brain two functional minds- a **Scientist Mind** in the dominant cerebral hemisphere of the brain and a **Spiritualist or subconscious Mind** in the other hemisphere. He got Nobel Prize for this concept. Edward De Bono also told the same thing in his twin hemisphere theory. Scientist Mind is in the left dominant hemisphere in the right handed persons. Psychiatrists believe that today there is nothing right with the left brain and there is nothing left the right brain.

Our mind is a double edged weapon. Scientist Mind is judgmental, logical, analytical, mathematical, always calculating and the seat of all the negativity in the form of negative thoughts, emotions and desires. In short it is the most powerful weapon for self destruction. It demands scientific proof for existence of an entity for believing and having faith. A mindset which is very rigid about the scientific proof is known as having **Scientism**. All the turbulence occurs only in this mind. It is responsible for Linear thinking which always tells two plus two is four only.

Spiritualist Mind has immense potential in terms of wisdom [vivek or saar-asaar buddhi], knowledge, power and experience of last several births. This mind functions on belief or Bhav and faith or shruddha. It is responsible for **Lateral or Out of Box thinking** in which two plus two could end up in infinity. The gut feeling or intuition or sixth sense or extra sensory perceptions, [E.S.P.] creativity and innovation are the novel qualities of this mind. Yoga-siddha have the super human powers of clairvoyance, levitation, miracles like walking on fire or water, astral form of travel, Para-Kaya- Pravesh and suspended animation because of extra-ordinary development of Spiritualist mind or Satvik consciousness by Kriya yoga.

Dominant mind makes **learning a very complicated process**. Remember when one is having car driving lessons. The constant flow of instructions confuses us so much that we push the accelerator instead of putting on the break. But once the learning by **linear thinking** process is over, spiritualist mind takes over and everything becomes easy and automatic. Meditation helps to inculcate moral and ethical values in this spiritualist mind. Once this process is over, value based life becomes automatic and easy.

Belief and faith are very important for health. Today, the patients have lost faith in the healing profession. This may also be one of the important reasons for rising incidence of incurable chronic diseases. A recent study in **Journal of consciousness** has shown that the placebos, non-medicinal substance curing a disease have become 70 to 300 times more powerful than the drugs. American FDA rule says that if placebo is even 30 times more powerful then the drug should be withdrawn. This rule has resulted in the closure of several drug manufacturing firms which marketed drugs for Crohn's disease, Schizophrenia and Depression.

NTELLECT AND WISDOM

Intellect is the ability of the mind to learn the skills for livelihood quickly.

Wisdom or Saar-asaar Buddhi or Vivek is very important because it gives the power to the mind for using the God-given intellect properly in accordance with the universal cosmic laws.

Spiritual vacuum or Adhyatmik shunyata is the term coined by Dr. N.N. Wig, an internationally renowned Psychiatrist and a Professor emeritus at PGI, Chandigarh. This confirms the importance of spiritual dimension of health included by **W.H.O. in 1998** in the definition of total or holistic health. Research in Mind Body Medicine has shown that the other three dimensions namely physical, mental, social or emotional dimensions could collapse any moment and that too very suddenly resulting in Burn Out or suicides.

Spiritual vacuum leads to lack of wisdom, or Vivek-shunyata or the loss of power of differentiation between right and wrong. **Today, nearly 18500 human genes** have undergone transformation giving human race that is extremely intelligent, an indicator of oncoming Golden Age. The previous I.Q. scales have become outdated. The genius level people by previous IQ scale come in lower five places by the new IQ scale. But unfortunately in Kali-yug or Iron age, the Devil, Shaitan, Ravana or Maya become very powerful. So these highly intelligent but wisdom less persons fall in honey trap, money trap or in both. Wisdom less state of mind leads to wrong pursuits in life, invites diseases, addictions and early march to the grave.

GENESIS OF TRAITS, [SANSKARA], HABITS,NATURE [VRUTTI, MINDSET] AND ADDICTIONS.

Research in Mind Body Medicine has proved that the positive thoughts [Sankalpa] are wonderful instruments of healing. But a negative mindset is sure to lead to diseases, addictions and early death.

A thought is responsible for giving us our habits, Nature, attitude, perception and behavioral pattern in the following manner.

A negative thought if formed repeatedly results in bad karma under appropriate circumstances. The inner voice shouts the loudest to prevent the crime or sin.

121

When repeated karma of same kind happens, it gives rise to habit. The inner voice gets feebler and feebler. A stage comes when a desire for **instant gratification** develops as the warning voice has completely disappeared.

A HABIT once formed is very difficult to remove. You remove H. Abit remains. Remove A. Bit remains. Now you finally remove B. It remains. So what is the solution to the problem of bad habit or addiction? Remove I or Ego which also means Erasing God Out of your life. This shall allow T or Transformation to happen. Regular practice of BK-Rajayoga for just half an hour reduces the I or ego to a remarkably low level within **three months**. When this happens, an individual gets the power of **samyak shravan** or an ability to listen to others with laser beam focus. He also gets a power of differentiation between right and wrong. In addition he develops a gut feeling about any situation and then he is able to chalk out the best possible course of action. He is able to ask the following questions to himself-

1] Is the given suggestion harmful to him in any way?

2] Are there any benefits for the self and what are they?

3] Is there any scientific evidence about the claims made by the person? Many a gullible persons could save themselves from exploitation by the quacks. The same applies to the BK-Rajayoga also. If the people ask the above mentioned three questions to the self, then they would come to a logical conclusion about any spiritual and yogic strategy for health and miracle cures.

4]   In what way BK-Rajayoga is different from more than two hundred different forms of meditation?

A HABIT of long standing duration results in the formation of our Nature, Vrutti, Prakruti or mindset.

Our nature decides the quality of our perceptions, attitude and behavioral pattern.

Nature once it becomes engraved in our psyche or subconscious mind, it gets transmitted to the next birth as Trait, Latencies or Sanskara or a spiritual genome.

Past Life Regression Hypnosis or Therapy [P.L.R.T.], child prodigies and re-incarnation studies have provided scientific proof for the Vedic truth that traits or karmic accounts are transferred to next birth.

A neonate having congenital heart anomaly undergoing immense suffering and pain also proves the truth in Karma theory of Bhagavad Gita. The bad karmic load of the past birth **[sanchit karma or prarabhda]** remains unfinished due to suicide or death by other unnatural means. Hence the Bhog starts right from the birth.

CHARAK SANHITA, CONSCIOUSNESS AND HEALTH

One thousand years old Charak Sanhita describes 15 types of personalities [Prakruti] depending on the consciousness as predominant the criterion. Three main types are Satvik [a soul conscious state of mind], Rajasik and Tamasik [Body conscious state of mind].

Satvik is divided into six types-

1] Brahma type – He is purest, devoted to truth, has extreme self-control, most knowledgeable and most powerful. He is capable of scientific, philosophical and religious discourses. He has good memory and has immense power of understanding. He is free from greed, conceit, intolerance, desires and infatuation.

2] Rishi type- He is devoted to vows, celibacy and sacrifice, has genius level capacity, eloquence and memory. He is devoted to contemplation.

3] Indra type- He is brave, energetic and authoritative of speech, endowed with splendor and possesses foresight. But he is given to the pursuit of wealth and sensual pleasures. Indra is the prototype.

4] Yama type- He is governed by the considerations of propriety, authority and is free from passion, attachment and has a good memory. Yama is the God of Death.

5] Varun type- He valiant, full of courage, intolerant of unclean surroundings, fond of aquatic sports and sacrifice of animals. He has well placed anger and fervor. Varuna is the deity that presides over cosmic order.

6] Kubera type-He commands status, honor, luxuries, wealth and is given to the pleasures of recreation. He is fond of singing, dancing, music and praise. Though addicted to the pleasure of women, fragrance and recreation, he is devoid of envy.

RAJASIK PERSONALITY

1] Asura type- valiant, terrifying, fond of self adulation, possesses authority and is pitiless.

2] Rakshasa type- cruel, gluttonous, intolerant, and full of hate. He is fond of pleasures of food and flesh. He is capable of biding time and then striking.

3] Pisacha type- eats voraciously, fond of secret company of women, hates cleanliness and indolent is disposition. He arouses fear in the beholder. He is fond pleasure of food and flesh.

4] Sarpa type- Touchy, indolent disposition, arouses fear in the beholder, and addicted to the pleasures of food and recreation.

5] Preta type- His character, pastimes and conduct are of painful disposition. He is covetous, envious, and disinclined to work. He lacks power of discrimination. They live on human corpses.

6] Sakuna [bird] type- constantly devoted to eating and sports, fickle and intolerant.

TAMASIK PERSONALITY

1] Pssva [animal] type- mentally deficient, disgusting in behavior and food habits, abandoned to sexual pleasures and has somnolent habits.

2] Matsya [Fish] type- cowardly, gluttonous, fickle, prone to quick anger and sensuality. He loves water sports and roving.

3] Vanaspataya [Plant type] – Very lazy and devoted to business of eating. His intellect is subnormal.

Ayurvedic treatment is based on three doshas- Vatta, pitta and kapha and on Prakruti or personality type.

POWER OF THOUGHTS

Mind boggling research on thoughts [Sankalpa] in the R & D institutes in Russia has recently come out in light after the disintegration of Russia. Why this unexplained disintegration suddenly happened? I believe that the karma theory of Bhagavad Gita gives an adequate explanation.

Faraday cage experiment in Russian research Institute identified three types of persons- Powerful thought transmitters, powerful thought receptive persons and the usual population. Faraday cage is novel. Nothing leaves this cage by any known scientific modes and means of transfer. **Thought transmitter** in the cage was given a log book to record the time and exact thought he transmitted. Thought receiver seated outside the cage also had a log book to record the time and messages he received. This experiment proved that our thoughts could be transmitted to infinite distance, even to and from USA. Russians then identified transmitting and receiving type of persons in children. They received special military training. All these young men were given only one task- to gain confidence of their superiors in various sensitive areas and to reach to the top most possible level where top secrets would come to them naturally. Process of transmission of top military secrets started. Democracy could only raise doubts but could never prove the existence of this nefarious activity because of the lack of evidence. Russia came to the verge of becoming the ONLY SUPER POWER in the world. But this was not in Divine Plan. The karma of interference in God's wish resulted in disintegration. USA then became the Only Super Power.

Faraday cage experiment proves the phenomenon called Telepathy.

Yuri Galer, a giant Russian, has a unique power of telekinesis. He could move the hands of the school clock and was a favorite amongst his school classmates for his unique ability. He came to Mount Abu, the International headquarter of a global N.G.O., known to the world as Brahma Kumaris. Only a few know that this unique N.G.O. has won six international peace awards. It also has a consultative status in U.N.O.**Dadi Janaki**,the Head of this global N.G.O. had been certified as the most stable mind in the whole world by two independent teams of neuroscientists in USA and Australia. Bhagavad Gita calls this state of mind as the state of spiritual equipoise or equilibrium [***Sthit-pragna avastha***]. Some manipulative Brahma Kumars brought the two unique persons on a stage. Yuri Galer performed his tricks. Dadi Janaki was then asked about her opinion. Dadi quietly told- Bachcha hai. Karatab dikha raha. A child is showing his childish tricks. Yuri then was asked as to what are his feelings now. He said he is feeling like a small child in front of giant Dadi. Surprisingly Dadi is not even five feet tall. Is this the effect of mesmerizing and powerful thoughts constantly emanating from Dadi Janaki? Scientist minds must investigate and tell to the world.

SCIENTIFIC EXPERIMENTS SHOWING UNBELIEVABLE TRANSFORMATION BY APPLICATION OF THOUGHT POWER

1] Mexican Neuroscientist, Dr Jacob Grinberg-Zilberbaun, in 1977 spent several months watching the mind boggling operations a Mexican psychic surgeon woman known as **Pachita** performed without anesthesia. She used a mountain knife and replaced diseased organs with healthy ones which appeared out of thin air. He admitted that his descriptions of her operations sounded like the ravings of a mad man. But science is an infant. It cannot grasp that such miracles could happen.

2] Backster effect-[February 1966]- Backster in CIA was involved in hypno-interrogation using polygraph machine. He began an intensive polygraph research on human beings. He connected his dracaena plant to the polygraph in his novel experiment. Surprisingly the plant showed the signs of life. It showed a jagged pattern of the live forms changing from moment to moment. It looked like the pattern of a person who was about to lie. He now tried to confirm if he can get a human like response from the plant by threatening its well being. He dipped one of the leaves in cup of hot coffee. Nothing happened to the chart. Then he merely thought when nearly fifteen feet away from the plant may be, he should burn the plants electrode leaf. At that very moment when the thought developed in his mind, polygraph recording pin moved rapidly as if the plant has read his mind. Backster repeated his experiment in front of his students. A student jumps out of his seat with a lighter in his hand and runs towards the plant to burn it. The plant screamed in the graph from the fear of getting burnt. Then the student told the plant he is sorry and spoke some words of love and affection. The graph calmed right back down.

Backster performed his experiment with human cells in 1988.He brought NASA astronaut and his friend **O'Leary** along with a lady friend to his lab. Backster obtained live cells from mouth scrapings of **O'Leary** and connected them to polygraph. In his laboratory, **O'Leary** and his girl friend had some violent argument and the graph gave high intensity response. Backster and O'Leary synchronized their watches and **O'Leary** then left to fly back to his home in Arizona. Next day the graph showed a precise correlation between the stressful events that happened on the way back, for instance- rental car missing the exact turn to the airport, stress of missing the flight and finally when his son did not show up at the airport to receive him. This shows that whole nature is in constant conversation with each one in it by as yet unknown mechanism. This has been called as **Universal mind** or all pervasive Universal consciousness and is also known as collective consciousness. The phenomenon of simultaneous discovery is another proof for the existence of universal mind. Dr. Medawar in England and Dr Burnett of Australia, in 1960, simultaneously discovered the subset populations of Thymic Lymphocytes. This brought on a tremendous impact in the field of immunology.

RIGOROUS LABORATORY PROOF FOR CONSCIOUSNESS TRANSFER

Dr. William Braud in 1960 attempted to transfer his thoughts to his one of his students while the student was under hypnosis. Braud pricked his own hand and the student felt the pain. When he put his own hand over a flame, the student felt the heat. Distance did not matter because the student was in her home many miles away. This is the proof that people could transmit their pain through their thoughts or they can heal you by sending comforting thoughts. However, as a protection by the nature, these thoughts cannot affect a person who is not willing to accept them. Hence the experiment is successful only in **hypnotized person**.

3] Lucid and Mutual Dreaming and Dream Telepathy - Dr. LaBerge-Sleep Research Centre-

Dr. LaBerge devised a technique called as Mnemonic induction of lucid dreaming [MILD]. This technique allows a person to wake up naturally and immediately after a dream. Salvatore Dali, a famous Italian painter, used to sleep with a spoon in one hand which was positioned to remain over a tin plate. No sooner REM sleep- [Rapid Eye Movement] or dream stage happened, the spoon used to fall on the tin plate waking up Salvatore. Then he painted the beautiful creation which he saw in his dream. These paintings are unique.

Bacteria, plants, insects, animals and all human beings all appear to be sharing the same mind [Consciousness]. Scientific breakthroughs all over the world consistently seem to happen in parallel. **Remote viewers** can make detailed observations of distant locations or create measurable signal of their presence in those areas. Shri Sai charitra of **Sai baba** of Shirdi mentions that Sai Baba remained in Shirdi and at the same time was present to partake in lunch at his devotee's place several hundred miles away. Now it seems there is a scientific evidence for such an unbelievable quote in Shri Sai Charitra.

Ancient Indian concept of Third eye [Spiritual eye or Divya chakshu]-

All of the religious philosophies give great importance to Pineal gland as "God's antenna" for receiving cosmic signals. Psychiatrists call it as God's spot as it now believed that pineal gland is the seat of the soul or atman. This tiny gland is roughly situated deep in the brain tissue in the axis that passes through the centre of the forehead. This information provides the scientific evidence to the BK-concept that soul, a metaphysical conscient point of light, exists in the centre of the forehead in between the two eyebrows. Pineal gland lying deep in the brain tissue and in total darkness has a structure like a human eye or retina with photosensitive rods and cones, piezoelectric and piezochromatic crystals and a fluid rich in DMT and melatonin. **DMT [Dimethyl Tryptamine]** resembles structurally Psychedelic or hallucinogenic drugs like LSD. DMT has tremendous piezoluminiscence. Piezoelectric and piezochromatic crystals are photoactive i.e. they are activated by light energy particles or Photons. All of these components take part in visualization like a human eye. This scientific information provides strength to the spiritual concepts in all the religious philosophies that pineal gland is meant for receiving cosmic signals. It is possible that the belief that pineal gland in God's messengers is exceptionally large is scientifically correct. Spiritual practices may enhance DMT production and may be responsible for the transcendental or deep meditative states. Thus one could experience LSD effects without any cost or side effects by meditation. Pineal gland is not protected by blood brain barrier. Secondly the gland accumulates fluorides rapidly for some unknown reason. This fluoride accumulation is detrimental to health. Electromagnetic radiations [EMR] from mobile phones enhance this fluoridification. Hence fluoride rich tooth pastes are also dangerous. Fluoride apparently passes directly into the pineal gland, and then gets attached to the tiny crystals in pineal fluid. Soon these crystals get covered with hard mineral deposits creating white bone like lumps in X-ray images. This pineal calcification is associated with grave health consequences. Fluoride interferes with the synthesis of Melatonin from melatonin precursors like serotonin and 5-methoxytryptamine. Melatonin controls the sleep wake cycle. So pineal gland calcification is evidenced by disturbances in sleep cycle and insomnia. Research has shown that this **sleep back log** is highly hazardous to health and may be an early cosmic signal for impending death. Melatonin is also associated with regulation of memory and cognition. These findings emphasis that melatonin has a specific role in the mechanisms of consciousness, memory and stress. Thus it may have a role in patients with Depression, schizophrenia, anxiety disorders, eating disorder like bulimia anorexia nervosa, tardive dyskinesia, Parkinsonism, epileptic seizures and other mental disorders. Painful conditions like gout may also arise. Teeth deformities and dental cavities may also be associated.

The most important prevention to pineal calcification is drinking lots of water throughout the day, may be 2 to 3 liters or more. The indication for adequate hydrotherapy is that the urine is always clear and like water. Avoid processed foods. Eating fresh organic raw food ensures that pesticides and food preservatives do not accumulate in your body. All of these measures may help to decalcify the pineal gland if its calcification has happened. Dr. Price identified a compound called Activator X or vitamin K-2 in traditional foods which is key ingredient. This vitamin K-2 is present in meats, eggs and fish. Dr. Price recommends Butter oil from cattle who feed only on fresh organic grass for the vegetarian persons.

ISKCON, a worldwide spiritual organization has such source of Indian cows that are fed on fresh organic grass. ISKCON now has Gaushalas with gaupalaks and gaurakshaks with a mission to save Indian cows from butchers. Indian cows at the most give 10 litres of milk per day and Jersey cows give a fantastic quantity of 50 litres per day. Poor farmer thus is forced to sell his Indian cows to meat processing multinationals. These cows are forced into a lorry and transported to meat factories in most inhuman conditions. There the cows are given an injection that swells them up. This is followed by another injection which removes the excess of fluid from the body. Muscles then get separated from the skin in most painful way. Half dead cow is then hung from a meat hook and a cut is given in jugular vessels to bleed the animal. Blood is used for haematinic preparations.

We Indians if we start believing in Karma theory in Bhagavad Gita while doing such cruelty to cows, we may stop doing this butchery altogether. As you sow, so you reap.

There is another strong reason for saving Indian cows. These are unique in that they have a hump on the back. This hump is believed to be condenser of cosmic energy. Thus the milk from Indian cows is most suitable as a diet as it contains all the proteins that are required by human beings in most digestible forms. In addition, probably this milk is charged with cosmic life-force. Only the milk of Indian cows in proper dilution is most suitable for infants if mother's milk is not available. In short it nourishes and in some unknown way sharpens the intellect and brain power. This may be the reason that India had the persons called as Ekpathy or Dwipathy with exceptional memory in yester years. This milk which is called as A-2 milk by ISKCON is thinner than that of Jersey cows. But it is very healthy. A study in New Zealand has shown that children there are getting heart attacks because of consumption of the jersey cows' milk. So save Indian cows and save yourself from heart attacks and allergies and deficient mind power.

Several Hindus are also beef eaters today. They must remember one mantra that tells as follows-

Hey mother cow whatever I am giving you in this birth by way of eating your flesh, I hereby authorize you to do the same thing with me in my next birth.

4] THE HUMAN CONSCIOUSNESS PROJECT-

Schlitz and Honorton [2004] explored thirty nine different studies during which people successfully shared their thoughts and experiences even while they were physically separated from one another in a different room or location. More than five hundred publications on SHARED INTELLIGENCE have proven that human consciousness can affect biological as well as electronic systems. Even when the participants were in separate rooms, their heart and brain waves became synchronized and they also felt appreciation, love and empathy towards each other. When the people were able to synchronize their heart waves and achieved Left and Right brain-waves coherence through meditation they caused heart waves and brain waves of the other individuals in separate room to become synchronized with their own pattern. Discovery of mirror neurons in the frontal brain proves the existence of a silent transpersonal exchange between the two individuals even though not a single word has been spoken. This phenomenon is responsible for the "Sixth sense", Gut feeling or "Intuition" about the other person. This subtle mechanism is well honed in the females and acts as a protective mechanism for them. An increase in the level of gut feeling could be so enhanced as to give the power of "Reading" the other person's thoughts or mind. Women are the best judge of a person about his nature [Vrutti]. BK-Rajayoga has been shown to produce greater coherence between the Right and Left brains thus enhancing empathy and **Emotional Intelligence**.

Dr. Braud found that participants in the research could increase the speed of running of gerbils by focusing on a single thought to that effect. They could also protect human Red Blood cells from lysis when put in a strong saline solution that immediately kills the cells. Dr. Braud and his associates could calm the nervousness and remove the inability to concentrate in patients with anxiety disorder by simply concentrating on them from another room. This provides a scientific proof for the concept of Manasa Seva in Brahma Kumaris spiritual practice. It has been also found that one can protect oneself from the impact of negative emotions on us by continuously maintaining a positive mental attitude. This is the scientific basis for divine protection conferred by Nirantar Yaad in BK-spiritual practice.

Dr. Deryl J. Bem [2011] showed by his research that human consciousness has direct access to the future. This proven scientific concept could substantiate the existence of **Turia consciousness** in which state the mind could see the past, present and future events in very precise way. This is known as Trikaal-darshi avastha or clairvoyance described in ancient Indian scriptures.

Dr. LaBerge concepts about the dreams-

The concepts believe that every landscape, every object, every character and every situation in the dreams represent some forgotten aspect of you. A dream is a message from your subconscious mind or astral body. The language of dream is symbolic. Every symbol is a part of some situation that is happening to you in your waking life For instance, if someone is abusing you in waking life, he may become a monster in your dream. Threatening, terrifying and aggressive characters in your dream represent some aspect of your own self that you have not forgiven or accepted. Dr. LaBerge technique teaches you to identify these situations as dreams and then to use them as triggers to become lucid and clear in your consciousness.

In a lucid dream, Out of Body Experience [OBE] or Near Death Experience [NDE], remote viewing session, hypnotic trance, or coma our subconscious or spiritualist mind may be using cosmic consciousness much more than when we are conscious. Predominance of Scientist Mind doing judgemental linear thinking is a common state of mind during wakeful state. So Edgar Cayce's readings may actually be quoting from the limitless cosmic consciousness after the scientist mind has been put to sleep by hypnosis.

A Czech motorcyclist was knocked out in an accident. When he woke up he started conversing in fluent English and he even forgot that he was Czech. However, within a short time he lost his new found ability.

A Croatian girl woke up from coma speaking fluent German.

David Wilcock began practicing Dr. LaBerge technique.

One day he stuck gold. In a lucid dream he could fly, levitate, walk through the walls and manifest anything you want to see or experience, even change the entire environment with a snap of a finger. Lucid dreaming means bringing whatever you have dreamt into physical reality. One day David was in a departmental store. He levitated over the whole series of big plastic garbage cans and started orbiting them around each other like a little solar system. Everyone in the store stood there in awe. Then suddenly he realized like a flash that he was dreaming. But the after experience was amazing. Vividness of life increased hundred fold. Even the common place items seemed alive and very beautiful. He felt absolutely well; clear brained and free. All these events may be happening in a deep meditative state.

Roger Levin in 1980- published – Is your brain really necessary?

Hydrocephalic children had only five percent of their regular brain tissue left. But several of these babies had I.Q.s greater than hundred.

A student at an American University gained first class honors degree in mathematics and was socially completely normal. A brain scan was performed for some health reason. Shockingly his cranium was filled mainly with cerebrospinal fluid.

DNA MEASURABLY RESPONDS TO HUMAN CONSCIOUSNESS-

Most coherent brain wave patterns have the strongest ability to change the structure of DNA in the genes. According one gene one enzyme hypothesis each gene is responsible for one specific feature in our body. In one experiment when DNA solution was placed in front of people who were generating right and left brain wave coherence by meditation, but not trying to change the DNA , there was no change in winding and unwinding of DNA in the sample. It is only when they wanted it to change that DNA actually did it.

In another experiment, Dr. Lew Childre was able to wind and unwind DNA in his laboratory from half a mile away by merely thinking about it.

Valarie Sadyrin was able to wind his own DNA in Dr. Rein's laboratory in California from his home in Moscow. According to Dr. Rein the key quality of the unknown energy that is generated by coherence in brain waves and could be transmitted to bring a transformation in DNA is love.

Both of these studies provide proof that positive quality of powerful thoughts could affect the unhealthy genes and bring about a repair from a great distance. This provides credibility to the Reiki concept that Reiki masters could heal a person from any distance. BK-Rajayoga also generated very powerful and positive thought vibrations. These could affect the unhealthy genes causing NCDs or Non-infectious Chronic Diseases and bring about an impossible cure. Meditation empowered mind could also be used for curing a difficult disease or addiction in near and dear persons by directing the thoughts of healing to the person.

It is possible that greater coherence of brain waves by meditation makes the energy-fields, nuclei and cells of our body to function in greater harmony and thus bring about Wellness. The coherent brain waves packed with emotion of love are most effective. Thus there is a lot of substance in the act of wishing well for others in the whole world. [Shubh chintan in BK-concepts] for everybody for the welfare of each one of us.

1] Peter Gariev study-[2000, 2001 and 2005]- Healing effect of coherent energy waves-

Laser beam is very coherent. Experiments from the year 2000 to 2005 consistently proved that a burst of coherent light can completely transform DNA molecule. Dr. Gariev poisoned a rat with alloxan to create alloxan Diabetes in which pancreas is completely destroyed. Then he removed pancreas from a healthy rat and gave a burst of green laser beam [healing] through them into the rat that had been poisoned. All the rats who received this treatment completely recovered. This could be the scientific basis for spiritual healing. Only thing that is necessary is developing exceptional power of concentration by meditative processes. This also provides a scientific basis for transformation of asuri or satanic Sanskara of another by a sadhak [spiritual practitioner] in BK-concepts. The coherence in our mind creates coherence in cosmic consciousness and in turn could affect everyone else's mind directly.

2] Gariev study- [2000]- Seeds died due to radiation in Chernobyl nuclear disaster were revived thoroughly simply by shining a non-burning green laser beam through healthy seeds on to the radiated dead seeds.

More surprisingly, all of these seeds grew into healthy adult plants.

In one case, Gariev was trying to grow a new healthy pancreas for a Diabetic woman by energizing her blood by shining the laser beam through the blood of her ten year old grandson. This is because the child's DNA still has the parents' and grandparents' Healthy "Energy Signature" in it. In just two weeks she started experiencing pain and swelling in her jaw. Soon new teeth cut through the skin. This forced the dentist to completely redo both her top and bottom dentures on account of new growth.

Dr. Gariev shone green laser through Salamander eggs on to frog's eggs and vice versa. Soon frogs hatched out of salamander eggs and salamanders came out of frogs eggs.

PSYCHIC ENERGY VAMPIRE-

Dr. Burlakov, a Russian scientist put more mature and older eggs in front of younger eggs that were just started in a hermetically sealed glass container more mature and older eggs in front of younger eggs that were just started. The older eggs apparently sucked the life force energy out of the younger eggs. The older eggs grew stronger and faster while the younger eggs withered. This may explain why people feel tired when in contact with the negative people. Burlakov put a slightly younger egg next to a slightly older egg. In this case younger eggs would adsorb life force energy from older eggs till the growth and development was at the same level as others. This may provide a scientific basis for Sangh-Yog in which life force energies of all are brought to same level.

It was also observed that if you feel drained you can replenish yourself by connecting with Supreme Father, ocean of power in a state of coherence with heartfelt genuine love [A BK-Rajayoga concept].

Dr. Kaznacheyev kept two hermetically sealed cell cultures in close contact with each other and infected one of them. When he shone light from the diseased cell culture on to healthy cell culture, the healthy cells mysteriously got infected with the disease. Further on he discovered that if two people remained in close contact with each other they soon developed a great facial resemblance with each other indicating that possibly a spontaneous DNA transfer also may occur.

GLOBAL CONSCIOUSNESS PROJECT-

Heal the world by healing yourself

When we contemplate over global consciousness two terms become important - Human Mass Excitability Index and Mass Mind Intention.

1] A scientific study published in the Journal of offender rehabilitation [1993] a group of seven thousand people gathered at three different times and meditated with the thoughts of love and peace. Within a few months, a worldwide reduction in all acts of terrorism by a phenomenal seventy two percent was recorded.

In other event violent crimes, murders and rapes decreased up to 23.6 percent.

As soon as such types of gatherings ended, the crime level started going up back again. This effect works by sharing the same mind or global consciousness. The effect was enhanced when there was right and left brain coherence. Right brain in the right handed persons lodges spiritualist mind or subconscious mind which is devoid of any negative thoughts or emotions.

It has been also proved that if even a very small number of amongst us move into the meditative state called as "Pure consciousness" with the thoughts of love and peace, there shall be less accidental deaths, less warfare and less terrorism. This provides a scientific basis for the BK- concept- Self-transformation for world transformation.

2] Dr. Hew Len's Ho"oponopono technique-

Ho"oponopono is a Hawaiian spiritual practice in which contemplation over love and peace for everybody is done. Dr. Len was posted to a very dangerous Psychiatric ward. Here the psychiatrists quit on a monthly basis. The staff went on sick live very often. The attendants walked with backs to the wall to prevent lethal attack from behind.

Dr. Len used his variation of the Mexican spiritual practice. He remained in his chamber completely isolated from the ward.He reviewed the patients' case files daily to prescribe medication or discuss treatment plan with his staff. After this routine, he would hold each patients file for some time in his hands and kept on saying-"I am sorry. I love you. Please forgive me over and over again.He took on their problems and pains as if they were his own and worked on healing those issues within himself.

Within a few months the patients who were shackled were allowed to walk freely. Heavily medicatated patients started getting off their medication. Lastly the offenders who had absolutely no chance of getting out were freed. Soon the staff began to enjoy coming to work. Absenteeism and turnover disappeared. Soon staff outnumbered the patients. Today that ward is closed.

In nutshell you can heal the other person by healing yourself. BK-meditation harnesses this technique of healing the self. BK-spiritual practice of wishing well for each and everybody in this world [Shubh-chintan, Shubh kamana and Shubh bhavana] thus could have a potential to create tremendous impact in our efforts for global brotherhood and global peace.

SOME WEIRD DISCOVERIES/ Phenomenon

1] Ciba-Geigi's weird technology of genetic transfer and evolution-[1989]-

This major chemical company patented a process that allowed them to cultivate new and extinct or original forms of plants and animals. The process is deceptively simple. They placed the seeds of an ordinary fern between two metal plates and ran a weak DC current through them for three days as they germinate. They were astonished to find that the fern had transformed into a formerly extinct species that has only be found in fossils from coal deposits. The extinct fern had forty one chromosomes instead of usual thirty six. That means a genetic transformation happened without participation of the chromosomes. This is also a blow to Darwin's theory of evolution.

Ciba-Geigy then tried the technique with wheat. The species reverted back to a much older and stronger variety. This new wheat could be harvested after only four to eight weeks. The original species of wheat required seven months.

They tried the process on 200 million years old spores that were found in salt deposits 140 meters deep in the ground. Simply zapping them with electrostatic field brought them back them to life even though nothing has been able to revive these spores. But soon company realized that these plants could put them out of business.

2] LUNG-GOM- Ancient yog-Siddha like Sage Patanjali had the powers of levitation, astral travel, clairvoyance and suspended animation. Tibetan technique of Lung – Gom is also a technique of levitation. Tibetan monks are able to go into a deep trance state in which there is maximum coherence. In this state they can run along in huge leaps at remarkably fast speed using their bodies in a way that completely defies gravity. Each leap leads them to thirty feet high and one hundred feet forward. Author Alexandra David-Neel has actually witnessed a Lung-gom pa or a monk skilled in this fascinating art in action.

3] Italian scientist Pie Luigi Ighina- harnessed the energy that passes between earth and the Sun using his novel instruments. He was able to purify any food when used one device called Elios to zap it. If this is possible then prasadam or the food prepared and eaten in remembrance of God must be able to purify it.

One of his devices could neutralize earthquake. Another device called magnetic stroboscope when powered up could create a huge hole the clouds. Ighina also discovered the profound nature of matter- The atoms do not oscillate but vibrate. His magnetic field oscillator was awesome. It could change the vibratory state of particles and transform the material itself. For instance, he set up his instrument in front of an apricot tree. He gradually changed the vibrations of the tree to that of an apple tree. After sixteen days apricot tree gave apples.

Bhagwat Gita, Karma Theory and Destiny

Om saha Na vavtu, saha nau bhunaktu saha viryam karvah vahai.Om Shanti….shanti……shanti Hee.

Dr. Mrugesh Vaishnav, the Founder Chairman of Spirituality and Mental Health Task Force of Indian Psychiatry society [2006 to 2008] has conducted workshops on Bhagavad Gita in disaster management. He says "Spirituality means personal views and behavior that shows a sense of relatedness to the transcendental dimension or to something greater than the self." True mental health is when an individual has harmony within and also has harmony with others. This is emotional or social dimension of Health according to W.H.O. [1998]. Bhagavad Gita, a five thousand years old Indian scripture describes several anxiety and depressive disorders and also gives the concept of totally and mentally healthy person. Arjuna was the first sordid case of Depression. When he saw Bhishmacharya, Dronacharya and Krupacharya on the battlefield, he lost all confidence of a Mahavir or of great warrior. Fears, doubts, hopelessness and helplessness engulfed him. The condition is not dissimilar to a medical student appearing for the final examination.[Examination syndrome]. Quick fix psychotherapy by Lord Krishna revived him and made him battle worthy. In life each one of us is Mahavir Arjuna. Each one's enemies are different. But the common thread is anxiety, worry, doubt, suspicion, fears, frustrations, stress and tension. Today, omnipresent and omnipotent Stress has become a major killer of the young because of the stress associated diseases or lifestyle diseases. Currently these are known as Non-infectious Chronic Diseases [N.C.D.]. N.C.D. means a non-stop CD of life full of pain, suffering, addictions and diseases. BK-sahaj Rajayoga is a simple remix of knowledge from Bhagavad Gita and Patanjali Kriya yog which guarantees conquest of ageing and diseases. Current research in Mind Body Medicine tells about the release of rejuvenating neuro-hormones, Sirtuins, from brain during this Mindfulness Based Stress Reduction Program giving the conquest over ageing. I got rid of seven stress born incurable diseases by diligent and regular practice of BK-Rajayoga for just half an hour daily. But my relatives and doctor friends do not listen and prefer to suffer in continuous vicious cycle of pain and diseases. This is famous "Abhimanyu syndrome." BK-Sahaj Rajayoga provides psychotherapeutic solutions to day to day conflicts, relationship issues and performance pressures. A spiritual equipoise [Sthit-pragna avastha] is achieved within three months of practice. Then the mind becomes very powerful. Impossible starts telling I am Possible. Incurable diseases and addictions disappear permanently. Sadhak [practitioner remains in perpetual bliss and health. This is Happiness Quotient [H.Q.] which very essential for health. Khushi jaisi koyee khurak nahi.

Religion and spirituality are different. Spiritualism is a part and parcel of each religion. But each religion differs in accordance with the God's Message that varies and was pertinent to human survival at that point of time. Conflicts amongst human beings arise when one religious sect tries to convert others to his beliefs and faith. So Religion means divisionism, ritualism, dogmatism, nepotism, fanaticism and finally terrorism. Spirituality means remembering the original qualities of the spirit or soul namely peaceful, loveful, blissful, powerful, pure and knowledgeful. It perceives each human as the creation by the Supreme Creator, All Merciful The One and The Only One. No wonder, Ken Wilber in Transpersonal Psychology talks about an Atman to Atman trans-human transaction which brings equality in dealings. Free of cost BK- Foundation course emphasizes and focuses on this point alone so that it becomes a permanent part of our psyche. The corresponding behavior then becomes an automatic and easy action [Karma]. Bhagavad Gita is a science of self realization. Outwardly scattered consciousness is brought inwards to focus entirely on the Self with a single pointed focus of thoughts. BK-concepts believe that in this state a Yogagni develops which burns out our bad karmic account [Volcanic Meditation]. BK Dr. Chandrasekhar and several others got rid of their ferocious cancer by this technique. Carl Simonton's Institute of Psycho-oncology [1978] harnesses the healing power of mind by a Mindfulness Program, a mind – body regulation by meditation involving a set of powerful and appropriate auto-suggestion and concomitant visualization brought about miraculous results. Twenty two percent were completely cured. Average survival rate became doubled. Bernie Siegel from Yale University followed the Simonton method and found that several of his "Twelve months to live" patients were permanently cured of cancer. He called these patients as "Exceptional Cancer Patients [EcaP]. Psycho-neuro-endocrinal Immunology [PNI] is a branch of Mind Body Medicine. This science functions on the belief that the cells of the immune system could be conditioned through the training of the mind. Immune system then becomes a "Circulating Mind" [Dr. Naras Bhat 1995].

KRISHNA AS A COGNITIVE THERAPIST

Bhagavad Gita teaches us the science and art of living. Arjuna developed cognitive inadequacy. Krishna provided a new framework for the coping behavior.

First step was self-realization. I am an immortal, indestructible, ageless, timeless and powerful soul. I never got this perception in entire clarity until BK-foundation course made it very clear to me in an easy language. I am not this Body. I wear this clothing to play my role in this eternal world drama. My apparel for the role has been chosen in previous birth in accordance with my Karma.

Second principle- I am not the doer but an actor and a puppet on a string in this world drama. This is Witness attitude- Sakshi Bhav. I myself have created the strings

150

by my karma of past birth [Karma Bhog and sanchit karma]. My destiny in this birth is the result of karmic account. BK-concepts tell us a very encouraging spiritual truth. There are two ways of shedding the bad karmic burden- one is by undergoing avoidable suffering and the other by burning out the bad karmic account in Yogagni by volcanic meditation. Then the music of life shall come out.

Third component-

Clear and precise perception about Karma Yog, Japa Yog, Bhakti Yog and Gyan Yog or Rajayog which means true knowledge about the Self and The God. Rest all leads to confusion. My sojourn of twelve different Paths taught me a lesson- BK-Rajayoga is ultimate and very precise. Incorporeal God Himself gives this easy and simple knowledge through mystical experiences to a spiritually evolved and enlightened soul, Dada Lekhraj, an internationally renowned diamond merchant. When he became a Messiah and started passing on the knowledge to his progeny, Brahma Kumars, he became renowned as Brahma.

Each soul passes through four different phases of Yog -

1] KARMA YOG- –

It involves self-determination, self-discipline and self dedication to follow the values in life and the Straight Path while doing one's designated karma, For instance- Doctors must focus on healing. The person should never succumb to any temptations, pressures, attractions, desires [Vasana] or circumstances. One should do his designated karma to the best of one's ability without any expectations of name, fame, dame and wealth [Nirapeksha Bhav]. Karma should be performed with a firm belief and faith that I am just an instrument in the hands of Supreme Consciousness [Nimitta Bhav]. In such a situation karma becomes ultimate in excellence and always results in success. Hinduism calls it as following a Path of Shreyas. Holy Quran calls it Sirat al mustaqim. Hinduism and Islam are the only two ways of life given to the humanity through mystical experiences [Sakshatkars] by incorporeal God to a human conduit. Doctors today recite Hippocrates oath like a parrot. But they are unable to practice according to the oath because of the lack of three Ds – self determination, self discipline and self-dedication.

2] JAPA YOG-

Bad karmic account in life brings a man in a situation in which he becomes helpless and develops hopelessness. [Dil-shikasta in BK-concepts]. A friend then comes along and tells to have a japa or chanting of Om Namo shivaya thousand times in a day for one month. One starts chanting with complete belief and faith in the friend's advice. But chanting is very fast because worry laden mind is running very fast. Supreme Father of all the souls then sees that this child of mine, who has lost the memory of his true identity, and always thought he is the doer, is now asking solace from Me, his True Father. So God mercifully provides the solution. This is the beginning of the process of developing belief and faith in God. The person now starts believing that chanting has liberated him from a most tricky situation.

3] BHAKTI YOG-

The belief and faith generated by the 'experience' of chanting, Japa yog, calms the mind. Now the chanting is slow with complete belief and faith. This is Bhakti Yog.

4] GYAN YOG OR RAJAYOG-

When the divine terms and conditions of completion of the Bhakti Yog get fulfilled, The Supreme Himself decides that my divine spiritual child must receive the true knowledge about the self and the God. This is Gyan Yog or Rajayog. BK-concepts take a step further as the precise directions for a methodical Yog [Shrimat through Daily divine Muralis] and spiritual effort [purusharth] come as if from the God Himself, incorporeal God Shiva.

In essence Bhagavad Gita could be summarized into four principles- 1] Discussion [Pariprashna], 2] proper nutrition and exercise [Yukta ahara and vihar] 3]meditation [Ekagra mana] done with devotion [Shruddha] and 4] Total Trusting surrender to the Divine and Supreme consciousness.

Bhagavad Gita also speaks a little about Patanjali Yog sutra and ashtang Yog- Yama, Niyama, Asana, Pranayam, Dhyan, Dharana, pratyahar and Samadhi.

Ashtang Yog assumed great importance in Dwaper Yug [copper age] and kali-Yug [Iron age] in which man loses his soul consciousness and acquires Body consciousness. Soul consciousness means all the dealings are based on an Atman to Atman communication. Golden age and silver era have men stabilized in the deity-like soul conscious state Body consciousness means focus on body which brings divisionism in the mankind. Perception then is body oriented- male or female, rich or poor, Hindu or Muslim, Indian or Foreigner and several such identities in which the fundamental Truth and the true identity become lost. Bhagavad Gita tells emphatically that all the troubles of mankind arise out of body consciousness. Western Medicine has totally body conscious approach. Sheldon divides human beings in three Morphotypes- ectomorph, mesomorph and endomorph. Being or Atman is not taken into account. Hence Hippocrates, Father of modern medicine, nearly four hundred years ago, lamented- "Of the greatest error today is that the physicians do not take soul into account for therapy." Indian doctors are committing the same mistake today.

Sage Patanjali Kriya yog became known to man in the beginning of Dwaper or the phase of Vedanta. Man lost all the connection with Supreme Consciousness and became a directionless and rudderless creature. He became an easy prey for the Devil or Shaitan. Supreme Creator cannot bear to see His beloved children in grip of Devil. Holy Quran mentions that Shaitan had challenged **All Merciful Allah** that he shall bring all of His children under his reign. But Allah has told that His true believers shall never leave Him. Further, the true believers shall survive and thrive. Non-believers in Devil's grip [Bhrushtmati] shall enjoy short lived pleasures and wealth and then perish in pain and suffering at the time final deluge [Kayamat].

Phase of Vedanta indicates that the consciousness has become contaminated with Vasana, Vikalpa, Vikara and Vikshepa. A bad experience in the past gets embedded in psyche and alters our perception, attitude and behavior with another individual. This negativity is known as Vikshepa.

Seepage and leakage of soul energy begins now due to negative and waste thoughts. Memory cannot remember Vedas told verbally. Physical strength also becomes less. Further deterioration in the eternal Time cycle [Kalpa] results in the worst scenario of Kali Yug or Iron Age. Ill health and weak body become the hallmark of Kali Yug. Kriya yog also became ineffective today as the human beings do not have time and inclination to practice Kriya yog. The main reason is that there is no will power [Manonigrah]. Supreme Soul tells that "Janha dil hai wanha will hai. Nahi to bahut mushkil hai. If there is will there is a way. Otherwise it is very difficult." Today there are two main causes of pain, suffering and diseases- Ye Dil Hai ki manata nahi and Ye Dil maange more. Mind does not obey. Mind demands more and more. Our Mind is a double edged weapon. Lord Krishna showed Virat Darshan as the ultimate weapon to convince dejected Arjuna to fight the battle. He showed that all the persons in front of him are already dead. He only has to perform a pantomime or ritual of sending his arrows. The arrows have already done their job. But after this televised vision, Lord told

155

Arjuna- "Ultimately please do whatever your mind tells you to do". Thank God, Arjuna made the right choice. Hence we remember him as the greatest of warrior against phenomenal odds.- eight aukshahani soldiers with him. Kauravas [asuri or satanic Vrutti] had eighteen aukshahani soldiers. But the One and The Only One with Arjuna made the difference. BK-concepts tell this universal truth in a simple fashion- eknamy economy.

BK- Rajayog gives ruling and controlling power over mind [Dil]. The man can stop the agile mind to remain focused on the present moment. This is known as Mindfulness.

KARMA THEORY OF TWO ALTERNATIVES

Every moment, event, circumstance or a person provides two choices for final karma-Right or Wrong. Secondly God goes on sending the same type of event or person in your life till you have learnt a lesson from it. This is what is known as "Experience or Anubhav". Each event or a person is a question paper set by The Supreme for split second micro-examination to test the Gyan or True knowledge you have imbibed from the Divine instructions in Murali. In this novel examination, you are an examinee as well as examiner and the event or person is a question paper. The result is realized by the self immediately. Spiritualist or the subconscious mind is the judge. This famous "Inner voice" tells you immediately if you have failed.

Right or wrong is not decided by any authority in this material world. It is decided by eternal cosmic laws governing the entire Universe. They are same for all the human beings. Ignorance of these laws does not protect you from the punishment. Principle is very simple. As you sow, so you reap. You shall get back whatever you have done to the other soul against his or her wishes.

If mind dwells on bad thoughts, a bad karma happens sooner or later under propitious circumstances. When the bad karma is repeated often then it forms your habit, nature and trait eventually. Repetition of Bad karma goes on adding to your Bad karmic Load. It may pass on to the next birth as Traits or a spiritual genome if the karmic account remains unfinished due to suicide or accident. A small child undergoing intense pain and suffering soon after birth by congenital anomalies or deformities is an excellent proof for the karma theory. Good karmic account gives health, happiness, harmony, peace, prosperity and success or all the good things in life. So God gives us a pen in our hands to write our own Destiny [Bhagya].

Out Body Experience, Re-incarnation, Child prodigy and Past life Regression Hypnosis provide proof for Bhagavad Gita concept of re-birth.

GREATEST ERROR IN SCRIPTURES

Krishna is the first prince in the Golden age. Incorporeal Shiva is the One who has told Bhagavatam. Humanity suffered and went on descending to a lower and lower level of consciousness through Treta Yug [Silver], Dwaper Yug [Copper] and Kali Yug [Iron]. This descent on the spiritual ladder is associated with weakness in physical, mental. Emotional, social, moral and spiritual dimensions of health The fifth era [Sangam yug [Era of confluence] is known as Purushottam Yug. God Shiva Himself descends on planet earth and only in India and gives precise directions for spiritual effort through a human conduit. This is the original mistake in Shrimad Bhagavatam. One must remember that Shiva Himself tells Gita to the mankind whenever Dharma turns into adharm. Krishna is the first person who transformed into deity like status by the knowledge given by incorporeal Shiva.

Powerful Ruling and Controlling Points [Bindoo], Karma Bhog and NCD's [Abhimanyu Syndrome]

God has thousand ways of punishing us. But All Merciful always gives love, rewards and encouragement.

Human Being is a BMSO- Body Mind Soul Organism. Only Body and organism belong to this physical world. Mind and Soul are metaphysical, transcendental and beyond the realms of physical world. Current research in Mind Body Medicine has given following branches of modern medicine-

1. Spiritual Medicine
2. Energy Medicine

Spiritual Medicine is further classified into the following main branches-

1]   Psycho-neuro-endocrinal-Immunology   [PNI] [Sheridan et al 1994]- Deleterious effects of the stress and neutralizing them.

2]   Psycho-oncology Carl Simonton – Harnessing the hidden but immense healing power of mind for cure of the dreadful cancer.

3]   Psycho-pharmacology- Placebos stronger than drugs

4]   Neurogenetics- Allen's Brain map, cerebral genes and karma Bhog.

5]   Transpersonal psychology- Atman to Atman transactions which is very important for Human Resource Development [HRD]

6]   Receptorology – Conquest over ageing, diseases and infections. Dream of disease free, infection free and addiction free society shall become a reality.

2]   Energy Medicine- aims for harnessing life Force Energy or Prana and correcting or restoring the Energy Signature of tissues for permanent cure. The unique signature gets damaged or distorted by trauma, stress, infection and pollution.

2.1] Kriya yog- [Patanjali ashtang yog, Indian Integral Yog]

Yama, Niyama, Asana, Pranayam, Dhyan, Dharana, Pratyahar and Samadhi are the eight components of Kriya yog. Regular practice [sadhana] promises conquest over graying, dim vision, ageing and diseases

Acupressure and acupuncture are powerful techniques for cure of the incurable conditions..

2.2]   Prolo-ozone therapy- This is available at BK-Medical wing, Mount Abu. [BK Dr Rahul Lakhotiya-083870955]

2.3]   Korean Spiral Therapy- Sania Mirza had miraculous cure. [Dr. Jatin Chaudhari- 09811286852]

2.4]   Radionics or Vibrionics- The therapy consists of homeopathy like pills which are charged with Energized water. Therapy acts by restoring the damaged "Energy

Signature" of the tissues. [Dr. Deepa Hoskote 09833052296]

2.5] Cytotrone therapy- [Dr. G.S. Nayyar-09741118867]
This machine creates "Energy waves" and directs it on the damaged knee or other areas. Low energy waves restore the "Energy signature" and promote cartilage formation.

High intensity waves destroy the deep seated metastasis of a cancer.

Energy medicine requires certain pre-requisites. The first and foremost requirement is total trusting belief and faith in the therapy and on the person giving the treatment.

Flynn effect- Studies have shown that nearly 18000 human genes have undergone mutation giving rise to a highly intelligent human race. Unfortunately intelligence is not supplemented by trusting belief and faith but skeptical mental attitude. In USA placebos have been found to be 70 to 300 times more powerful than the actual drugs used for treatment. This has shut the business of several pharmaceutical companies. American FDA is very strict. It discontinues all the drugs if placebos show even thirty times more effect than the drug.

Black magic and voodoo deaths depend on the belief and faith of a person that these tantrik methods do have a power to destroy him. In addition if he knows the person individually and believes that this person has the power to damage then deleterious effects happen with certainty.

Modern Medicine does not believe and does not have any knowledge about metaphysical entities which are beyond the grasp of modern scientific technologies. This disbelief is simply because a scientific proof is absent about the existence of these entities. This is unfortunate because it prevents the mainstream medicine from investigating and proving the truth about the claims of miraculous cures by alternative therapies. This rigid mindset of modern mainstream medicine keeps open a huge area for exploitation of the gullible by the quacks. Even in USA 84% of the persons opt for alternative therapy because of sky rocketing cost of modern investigations and interventions. In end stage terminal cases like cancer or AIDS, the figure rises to astronomical 94% approximately. USA FDA has declared Radionics as Pseudoscience. But several American institutes are conducting courses and issuing Diploma for Radionics.

AYUSH – Ayurveda, Yoga, Unani, Siddha yog and Homeopathy is doing a silent but tremendous job of providing relief to the masses in the healthcare by using ancient art and science of healing. Mainstream medicine looks upon it with contempt and takes satisfaction in celeberating Anti-quackery day on first of July, the "Doctors" day. This certainly is an unhealthy response and an exercise in futility.

The following powerful Points control and rule over all the physiological and biochemical functions of a Human

Being or Body Mind Soul Organism [BMSO] . Only some of the Points have been demonstrated and more importantly accepted by the medical science.

A] METAPHYSICAL POINTS AND PHENOMENA-
God, Soul, Energy chakras, acupressure and acupuncture points, Body aura, Cosmic Healing Vibrational whisper and Five body sheaths - Annamaya kosh, Pranamaya kosh, Manamaya Kosh, Gyanmaya kosh and Annamaya kosh and body aura.

B] PHYSICAL POINTS-
1]Cerebral centers- Reward and punishment centers, Hunger center, Satiety center, Sex center, Thirst center, Hypothalamus and mid brain nuclei and several others.
2] Genes- Cerebral genes, Somatic Genes, sex genes, oncogenes
3] and receptors.
Each point is so powerful that it can make life or destroy it by congenital anomalies, intractable genetic diseases, degenerative diseases or lifelong insufficiencies like Vitamin B-12 deficiency or Thalassemia.

A] METAPHYSICAL POINTS
God and soul have been dealt in details in previous chapters. We shall focus on other metaphysical Points.
1] Energy chakras-
Human Being has seven energy chakras from top to bottom- Sahasara, Agya, Vishuddhi, Anahat, Manipura, Swadhishthan and Muladhar chakra. Concepts by Alchemy of God by application of Sacred Geometry

have shown that cosmic energy [Life Force Energy] flows into various tissues through these metaphysical distribution points. Sahasara chakra energy is transcendental. It also supplies energy to Central Nervous system. Agya chakra in the centre of the two eye brows [Third eye or spiritual eye] supplies energy to Pineal and pituitary glands. Thus it takes part in controlling the various biological and biochemical processes in the body. It is believed that the Agya chakra is a central point in the zone of infinite positivity. Hence in BK-Rajayoga if the consciousness sways right or left or any where , it always lies in the positive zone. In Hath Yog or Kundalini awakening, the process of spiritual evolution begins at Muladhar chakra. This energy wheel lies at the center of infinite negative zone on one side and infinite positive zone on other side. Thus effects , both good or bad happen very fast. If the consciousness sways into negative zone then the person commits rape and murders. This may mean a huge bad karmik account that shall be needed to burnt out in one or more births. Vishuddhi chakra in the neck supplies thyroid and tissues in the neck. Anahat distributes energy to chest organs, Manipura to Gastro-intestinal tract, Swadhishthan to genito-urinary organs and Muladhar supplies genital organs. The energy flow from cosmos is called as Cosmic Healing Vibrational Whisper [Naras Bhatt]. Dr. BK Dr. Chandrashekhar, by an ingenuous use of Universal scanner demonstrates the body aura and the blocks in the chakras if present. The blocks in any chakra indicates and forewarns about an impending disease. Similarly the distortion and change in color of Body aura also is an early indication of the onset of a disease. All of these surmises need to investigated thoroughly by the mainstream medicine using their state of art equipments.

2] Acupressure and acupuncture points-
Dr. Robert Becker, an orthopedic surgeon studied the human body's natural electrical fields. He found that each and every person he strongest electrical field precisely at the acupressure and acupuncture points or Chinese meridian points.

A book by Marshal Govindan – entitled Kriya Babaji and eighteen yog-Siddha mentions that the first Yog-Siddha, Boganthar got the cosmic inspiration and he went to China to relieve the suffering of masses by his acupressure and acupuncture therapies. Thus the word Chinese acupressure may be a misnomer.

3] Body sheaths [Charak sanhita]-
Sukshma sharir or the Being is surrounded by five body sheaths from outside to inside- Annamaya kosh, Pranamaya Kosh, manamaya kosh, Gyan-vigyanmaya kosh and the inner most Anandmaya kosh. It is noteworthy that all the drugs in modern medicine including those used for mental disorders act only up to superficial most Annamaya kosh. Pranayam removes the impurities in Pranamaya kosh. Meditation removes the impurities in Manamaya kosh. When all of the koshas are pure and clean then soul enjoys bliss-anandmaya kosh.

4] Body aura-

Soul or Atman is a powerful transmitter of an electromagnetic energy in the form of vibrations. These vibrations around the body give rise to Body aura. Kirlian Body aura photography has demonstrated the existence of body aura. But world renowned clinicians and authorities like Padmabhushan Dr. R. D. Lele call it as an artifact. S.P.A.R.C. wing of Brahma Kumaris has a state of art aura scanner which shall be of great help in demonstrating the effect of deep meditative states on Body aura. In fact, the changes in or the distortion of aura is supposed to be earliest indication of impending disease of an organ. Immediate dismissal of Body aura as an artifact is the greatest impediment in bringing out a meaningful research to confirm or disprove such wild claims.

B] PHYSICAL POINTS

1] Cerebral centers-

These centers control and have a ruling power over hunger, thirst, satiety, sex and emotions.

Existence of Reward center, Punishment center, and Reverberating circuits in brain prove that Supreme Intelligence has provided an inbuilt mechanism to ensure good karma from the human beings. Whenever a man performs good or philanthropic karma he feels very good. This is because the activation of the reward centre releases "Feel Good Hormones" from the brain. On the other hand, when a bad karma is done "inner voice in Gyan-vigyanmaya kosh" shouts the loudest warnings. At the same time the punishment centre is activated. This releases detrimental stress hormones from the brain. Persona may be happy outwardly. But his innards are gnawing at him. This is the famous "Guilt conscience." Both of these good or bad effects remain activated for a long time because of the "Reverberating circuits."

2] Somatic and sex genes-
According to "One gene one enzyme concept" by Beadle and Tatum each gene is responsible for one specific function or feature in human body. Absence or mutation in any one gene produces profound manifestations. For instance- sickle cell anemia, Diabetes, Heart disease or genetic malformations..

Oncogenes- More than 200 oncogenes have been discovered. Each such gene is responsible for one particular form of cancer. Karma theory explains why one person gets a mild non-metastasizing cancer and others acquire virulent and rapidly lethal forms of cancer. Our karma doles out the pain and suffering in exact and precise proportion.

End stage battle of the soul-
Supreme intelligence has an unknown mechanism for keeping a precise and infallible record of the sins performed by the human beings. Hinduism believes that this record keeping is done by Chitragupta. Islam tells about two angels [Farishte] sitting on our shoulders and keeping the exact count. Kayamat is always different for different human beings. At this point of time Allah The All Merciful becomes a stern judge. Final judgment is by

three kinds of proofs-. First the angels read out the record. Modern intelligent man tells Allah that these witnesses have been purchased. Allah then shows the reel from eternally running CC TV camera. Man tells Allah that the film has been morphed. At this point of time the very organ by which the sin was committed starts giving its statement. Sin is then proved beyond doubt.

Recent studies have shown that average lifespan of an Indian has been prolonged by 20 years due to modern treatment. But all of these bonus years are spent in pain, suffering and diseases in an old age home or a Geriatric ward. The Quality Of Life QOL] becomes a victim. Energy, Enthusiasm and Happiness value [E.E.H. value] takes a back seat. BK-concepts explain these sad happenings or Karma Bhog in life on the basis of karmic load. The present birth is the last one for all of us. So the karmic load of previous births on us is very huge. The load or Karma Bhog could be mitigated by intense volcanic meditation in the present era known as Sangam Yug or era of confluence. Suli par chchadana tha to kaante par nibh jayega, ya fir kanta bhi nahi lagega. Karma bog could invite very severe punishment. But by intense meditation it could be neutralized. I believe that my emancipation from seven incurable diseases is because the specific karma Bhog has been neutralized.

In the light of the knowledge about karma Bhog it becomes very clear that our health and happiness in the present times may be the result of our accumulated Good karmic Account of the past births. But in this process our Good karmic Account is getting depleted. At the same we should be worried about the remainder of bad karmic Load which brings about sufferings in the end before our pre-ordained time of death. This is the famous End stage battle of the soul at the time of final reckoning or kayamat. In iron age bad karma happens in spite of careful watch because of the micro-forms of Maya. We may not identify them and subtly add to bad karmic Load. BK- concepts through Muralis tell us that if an uninterrupted remembrance [nirantar Dhyan] is done then yogagni shall mitigate sufferings before death. My personal experiences have helped me to develop firm faith in this spiritual concept. BK-Rajayoga technique is such that nirantar Dhyan becomes very easy. I now believe that by intense spiritual effort under Shrimat or Divine guidance as is available in BK-centres shall guarantee a painless death in which the breath and soul may leave the body in a second. The cry for euthanasia should be an indicator that end stage battle of the soul may be associated with unbearable sufferings. Regular practice of BK-Rajayoga at Amrit-vela or 4am for one hour has given me a life full of energy, enthusiasm and happiness [E.E.H. Value] at the age of 73 years. Supreme Soul in His Divine Muralis stresses often that Bhakti yog means the knowledge about the Supreme Sadgatidata is absent. Hence the benefits are obtained only for one birth. But Rajayoga gives the benefits for 21 births as the remembrance of the real

God, The One and Only One, is done with single pointed focus of thoughts. Life full of EEH value for 21 births may be a bonus. One must have the faith and belief about this guarantee from the Supreme Soul Himself. So I am making all the efforts to increase the duration of Yaad in my daily chart from 3-4 hours to 8 hours as prescribed by the God Himself. In fact whatever spiritual effort is done in Sangam Yug[era of confluence] , the beneficial effects last for whole of one time cycle[Kalpa]. I can make firm statement like this because of my personal experience. Even in the present phase of time cycle when I did not know about BK-Rajayoga, myself and my family were protected from severe harm while working at Ambajogai in Swami Ramanad Teerth rural medical college. I was told i am under double saade saatee- double wrath of Shani dev. Myself and my family came out unscathed and unharmed.

So I am doing my spiritual effort to the best of my abilities. The readers have to decide for their choice of action. Believer shall survive and thrive. Rest shall perish in pain and sufferings. Ancient Kriya yog promises wit, vitality and vision till last breath. But my personal experience is that the process is lengthy and time consuming. It is well beyond the capacities of modern Extremely Busy Persons [EBP] who forget that EBP also means an Easy way to high BP and heart attacks. BK- Sahaj Rajayoga is tailor made for the modern man who is always under time crunch.

3] Cerebral Genes-

Allen's brain map has discovered certain cerebral genes. The study of these genes is known as Neurogenetics. These cerebral genes remain quiet in happy and peaceful state of mind. But in stressful states of mind these dangerous genes get activated and release powerful enzymes. These enzymes in turn activate the somatic genes for various diseases. Thus ever peaceful and blissful state of mind goes a long way in maintaining our health and avoiding deadly diseases. BK-sahaj Rajayog gives this peaceful and blissful state within minutes after three months of regular practice.

Dr. David Eddie, cardiac surgeon in Stanford University did a research with Archimedes model which gave a virtual depiction of all the physiological and Biochemical functions in human being. The aim was to determine the increase in life span and benefits accrued from modern therapy. The results were shocking. Trillions and trillions of dollars spent on expensive investigations and treatment increased the life span by a mere three percent. The rest ninety seven percent came from proper sleep, sanitation, nutrition and a tranquil state of mind. Research has proved that deprivation of sleep and sleep back log is highly detrimental to health. Insomnia or sleeplessness is the earliest sign of impeding death. So the modern therapists now talk about sleep hygiene. BK-Rajayoga releases Melatonin, a neurohormone controlling sleep wake cycle and emancipates from sleeplessness. This open-eyed meditation has another unique feature. The meditation could be carried out for prolonged periods without the danger of falling asleep. Close eyed meditation has a very serious danger of person passing into Yog-nidra. After all modern man is always mentally tired because of his monkey like agile brain. When BK-Rajayoga is extended for adequate time, several regular practitioners show delta brain waves of deep sleep in E.E. G. studies even when the eyes are open. A practitioner of five years or more also shows the phenomenon of alpha blocking. That means he remains aware about his surroundings but does not get disturbed by external disturbances. A shield develops to involuntarily block unnecessary sensory perceptions. This quality is of great help in achieving the spiritual equipoise or Sthit-pragna state. Dadi janaki of Brahma Kumaris is the living example of having attained this feat. A study involving Kirlian Body Aura photography with Gas Diffusion Visualization shows that the body aura of Dadi Janaki goes beyond the recording plate with deepening stages of meditation.

4] Receptors-

These tiny Points on each cell of the body are unique. Bacteria, Microbes, fungi, enzymes, hormones, carcinogens and auto-antibodies cannot produce any effect until they are attached to a specific receptor. So a wonderful hypothesis has come into existence which needs to be investigated. If these receptors could be inactivated or made insensitive then the dream of achieving a disease free and infection Free states could become a reality. Receptor Modulation Factor [R.M.F.]

released during mindfulness gives the hope that the dream could become a reality very soon.

Stem Cell Activation Factor [SCAF] released during Mindfulness gives hope that all the degenerative disorders could be permanently cured. There are reports that five cases of fatal cardiomyopathy type b have been completely cured. Similarly three cases of partial blindness due to incurable macular degeneration have regained their complete vision.

God is creating miracles today. Man must have unshakable belief and faith.

NON-INFECTIOUS CHRONIC DISEASES [N.C.D.]

Latest terminology calls the stress associated modern lifestyle diseases as NCDs. The list of NCDs in the textbooks of Medicine is ever increasing. Spiritual Medicine shall mention only those which have assumed great importance and cause a virtual hell in life.

1] In children and adolescent- Obesity and Attention Deficiency Hyperactive Disease [A.D.H.D.] are important. Ninety percent of children with ADHD grow as adults with agile mind. Soon they develop Burn Out syndrome or develop addictions or end their life by suicide.

Alveolar hyaline membrane disease in infants is one in which the child drowns in its own secretions in lung.

2] In adults- List is very long-for instance Diabetes, Dementia, heart attacks, cancer and others. Interstitial Lung Disease [ILD] is so dreadful that in last fifteen years whatever newer drugs that have been discovered

173

reduce the lifespan of the person by half the expected time of survival. This Mehmood disease makes the person to carry his oxygen cylinder on the back and makes him suffer for five years until death emancipates him. Ramdeo baba's Pranayam and BK-Meditation has completely revived an Indian doctor's wife in USA. But Indian doctors treat Ramdeo baba and his yogic techniques for health with disdain. Thomas Babington Macaulay is having the last laugh even today in his grave.

Baldness-Alopecia-Marriageable young men develop inferiority complex and submit themselves to expensive and painful hair transplant procedures and invite pain in their lives. Cosmetic surgery is another means of inviting pain for interfering with God's plan. Botox injections for beauty are an indication of wisdom less vacant mind. Million dollar cosmetic and deodorant industry runs on giving a false hope of having a better face and refreshing breath to those persons who are not satisfied with what God and bad Karmik Account of past birth has given them. Stabilizing oneself in Soul consciousness by BK-Rajayoga, Satvik vegetarian diet, regular exercise, Pranayam and good thoughts may give emancipation from Acne or even halitosis or bad breath. But everybody desires a quick fix.

Obesity - forces young people to undergo expensive and dangerous bariatric surgery.

Addictions - have attained dangerous proportions.

Burn Out syndrome - This High achiever's syndrome exhausts all of the God-given stock of neurotransmitters and then he completely loses interest in life. This is the Burn Out.

Geriatric homes or wards- show a horrifying truth about modern lifestyle. Older people now get perceived as a burden and are quickly packed off to an old age home. These unfortunate people then start counting days before death shall show mercy and take away all of their troubles. Terrible disappointment that comes from lack of love and care makes the life hell for them. No wonder there is clamoring going on for euthanasia. Pet dogs become their sole emotional support in their lonely homes. But this emotional support comes with a heavy price. Numerous zoonotic diseases could get transmitted in the process.

Hinduism has a solution- Vaanprastha avastha. This involves asteya and aparigrah which means withdrawing one's consciousness from wordly affairs which never permit and getting focused on Supreme. The greatest hurdle in accepting this lifestyle is the ego and attachment to worldly affairs. They never permit detachment.

Secondly, TV mania make them choose a source of temporary and imagined happiness in place of a genuine and guided spiritual effort and spiritual evolution which guarantees everlasting peace, happiness and harmony. Empty hours are then spent on contemplation of the joys and sorrows of the characters in the TV serial. This loss of wisdom has become rampant in this Iron Age. Each one in a family wants his or her own TV as the likes and dislikes are different.

Power of adjustment is absent. Please never forget that all the years after the age of sixty are the bonus years for you. So it is wisdom to spend maximum time for shedding the bad karmic load to mitigate the end stage sufferings.

Various Infectious Chronic Diseases [N.C.D.S]

- ADHD Child
- ADHD Adult
- Obesity Child
- Obesity Adult
- Depression Child
- Depression Adult
- Burnout child
- Divorce
- Alzhemers
- Chronic Fatigue Syndrome
- Cancer
- Oncogenes
- Diabetes
- Alcoholism
- Smoking
- Multi tasking
- Information Highway Stress
- Stress Hair Loss Frustration
- Nagging
- Selfie Syndrome
- Road Rage Syndrome

Gods Pharmacy and Conquest of Greying, Ageing, Dim-Vision, Infections and Diseases

Supreme Creator has created a super duper car with all the protective, healing and curing mechanisms. Mind Body Medicine tells that the term **Healthy means Heal Thy.**

Recent studies have shown that live forms could **rewrite their own genetic code.**

Rockefeller University study [2009] showed that a parasite Trypanosoma brucei, cause of African sleeping sickness could spontaneously rearrange its own DNA so that it could not be detected and destroyed by body's defense mechanisms.

Nature always finds a way to repair the damage. Press release from Rockefeller University informed that even human beings could rearrange their DNA and get cured of a disease or intractable infection.

Dr. Robert Pruitt [2005], Purdue University, created a mutation in a plant in such a way that the plant developed flowers in an odd misshapen way. Subsequently even though the plants inherited genes from both parents, fully **ten percent of them reverted back to normal**. Scientists confirmed that the plant's DNA had undergone spontaneous mutation to rewrite and fix the damage. This was a critical blow to DAWINIAN MODEL. Somehow the genetic code of the plant was able to **intelligently rebuild the missing genes and corrected the damage.**

Dr. Dzang Kangeng [1993] found that he could transfer the genetic code from one species to another through nothing more than an energy wave. **A duck was placed in a pentagonal container.** Each of the five sides of the container had a hole with a funnel mounted in it. Each funnel had a pipe that fed into a neighboring room where there was a pregnant mother hen. The duck was zapped with a high frequency electrostatic generator for five days. Amazingly when the eggs from the hen hatched there were no baby chicks. They were **half-duck and half chicken hybrids.**

Italian scientist **Ighina** created a device called stroboscope for harnessing an energy that passed between the earth and the Sun., or an energy device that **could change the vibratory state** of particles and bring about the transformation of the matter. He altered the Vibrational state of the tail of a rat to change it in four days into the tail of a cat. He then excited the atoms of a rabbit's fractured feet. They were healed in a record time. Thus he hypothesized that the sick cells may be of cancer or Beta cells in Diabetes could be made normal by a gradual alternation in their Vibrational index.

Cosmic healing Vibrational Whisper created during Mindfulness passes through the energy chakras is also an unknown electromagnetic type of Vibrational energy. BK Dr. Chandrashekhar and several cancer patients in the series by Carl Simonton and Bernie Siegel became cancer–free by the mindfulness program. That means BK-Rajayoga, a mindfulness program has a potential to bring about impossible cures. This hypothesis needs to be investigated by meaningful research in Medical Institutes. The dictum of Mind Body Medicine– "Incurable disease means whose cure lies within" appears to have a lot of truth in it.

MIRACLE HORMONES RELEASED DURING MINDFULNESS MEDITATION

Inner silence oriented Mediations like BK-Rajayoga result in Ekagra Chitta avastha or Single pointed focus of positive thoughts.

Dr Herbert Benson, an American cardiologist and the founder of the first Institute of Mind Body Medicine tells that Meditators develop a state called as "Biological Relaxation Response or BRR and the Zone". This is indicated by a feeling of lightness and complete relaxation of the body and mind. This is an indication that Ekagra chitta avastha has been attained. This state of mind and body elicits ultradian rhythm of the brain releasing rejuvenating neuro-hormones. Normally this rhythm sets in after every 90 minutes. Hence a man can continuously work for just one and half an hour with full attention. After this time period he has to get up, go to the wash room or take a coffee during which time ultradian rhythm brings about recharging.

When Sunil Gavaskar in the Port of Spain scored 200 runs against the intimidating fast West Indian attack, he was asked how he could do it when other batsman were leaving their wickets open, he answered "I was in

the zone. I saw nothing else but the ball coming to me."
He was like Arjuna doing Matsya bhed, who saw nothing but the eye of the fish.

Studies have proved that brain releases several rejuvenating and healing hormones during the state of BRR. They are as under-

1] Encephalin-

This neuro-hormone restores the internal balance of lipid, sugar and ions. Thus possibly may bring about a cure of Hyperlipaedimia, Diabetes or High Blood pressure. Secondly, it gives a "Reverse Transport of cholesterol "from the lipid deposited in coronaries back into the circulation. This may be one of the factors in Coronary artery disease regression in Mount Abu Open Heart Trial initiated by President Abdul Kalam in 1998.

2] Endorphin-

It is a natural mood elevator and powerful pain-killer. The pain in terminal cases of cancer is not alleviated by any of the available pain-killers. But surprisingly practitioners of Vipassana or Maharshi Mahesh Yogi's Transcendental Meditation[TM] could bear the pain comfortably. Hardiness of mind or mitigation of pain by endogenous endorphin may be responsible for such situation.

3] Melatonin-

It is a secretion from pineal gland, the third eye [Divya chakshu]. It controls the sleep-wake cycle and is responsible for circadian sleep rhythm which is tuned to sunrise and sunset. Jet lag means disturbance in this rhythm. That is why frequent jet fliers suffer from a sleep back log which is bad for health. BK-Rajayoga elicits delta waves of deep sleep even when the eyes are open. Thus complete recharging is brought about by the Meditators.

4] Brain Derived Neurotrophic Factor- BDNF-
This neuro-hormone discovered in 2003 is blow to the theory that brain cells never regenerate. BDNF gives rise to neurogenesis and may prevent senile and other forms of Dementia.

5] Receptor Modulation Factor- RMF-
This factor released during Mindfulness makes the receptors on the cells of the body insensitive to the action of bacteria, viruses, fungi, auto-antibodies, stress hormones, Bacterial and fungal toxins, and to the enzymes released from cerebral genes. Thus this RMF could make the dream of infection less state and a disease less state turn into a reality. RMF could be the best answer to the problem of super bugs which makes the antibiotics useless for therapy. The stress born NCDs could have an easy free of cost solution for permanent cure.

6] Stem Cell Activation Factor-[SCAF].
Today the stem cells are grown in laboratory from fetal cells from umbilical cord for the stem cell therapy. These stem cells are then injected in the diseased part-

for instance damaged heart in infarction or knee pain due to damaged cartilage. But this advanced therapy does not guarantee cure and may have side effects.

Stem cells are totipotent cells. This means they could grow into any type of tissue- for instance heart muscle, cartilage or liver. Each tissue in the body has these stem cells. Stem Cell Activation Factor [SCAF] released during Mindfulness could activate the stem cells in the damaged area and could bring about complete recovery and rejuvenation. Till now, five case of cardiomyopathy type b and three cases of partial blindness due to macular degeneration have been completely recovered. This is a medical miracle.

7] Sirtuins-

Recently discovered Sirtuins make it possible to have the conquest over ageing. Patanjali Kriya yog promised the conquest of ageing. That means a person could retain his wit, vitality, vigor and vision till the last breath by a regular abhayas or practice of Kriya yog. Discovery of Sirtuins give scientific validity to the claim of conquest of ageing by Kriya yog prescribed by sage Patanjali 2500 years ago. Several books have come forth which are proving science behind Vedic concepts and those in Holy Quran. No wonder Scriptures teach us the true art and science of proper living. Sirtuin-2 is highly effective in retarding ageing.

8] Gut Like Protein-1 [GLP-1]and Gut Like Protein-2 [GLP-2]-

These proteins normally get secreted from the stomach wall and are responsible for satiety after food intake by their action on Satiety centre in the brain. The secretion of these proteins may get enhanced during mindfulness meditation and may prevent craving for food in Diabetes and other gut disorders like Bulimia.

BK-concepts talk about God in this way- Teri Gat mat bahut nyari. That means the ways of God are novel and a class apart. Till today we have discovered only seven of the miracle drugs in God's pharmacy. It is possible that many more might be in store to be discovered. Then we may believe in the eternal truth that the Golden race in Golden age has Kanchan Kaya which today is perceived as mythological fantasy. So it is a better choice of action to believe and act rather than waiting for the infant science to discover and prove that BK-Rajayoga is the panacea for all the ills that are plaguing the mankind today.

Yogasana for Health and Rehabilitation

Yog is a methodized effort [Purusharth] towards self perfection.

 Sir Arabindo

Book entitled "Kriya Babaji and 18 Yog Siddha" by Marshall Govindan mentions that Sir Arabindo was probably the last amongst yog Siddha. There is a story that tells about astral travel by Sir Arabindo. Neil Armstrong was hurtling towards moon in his spacecraft. He suddenly saw a beam of white and bright light emanating from earth and going into cosmos. When he plotted the location, the beam was coming from Sir Arabindo Ashram, Pondicherry. Sir Arabindo had isolated himself in a room for sadhana [spiritual practice]. So it is surmised that Sir Arabindo was undergoing astral travel in the form of beam of light. Mr. Govindan, a Canadian who took the surname from his teacher in KRIYA YOG also mentions that shiv lingams have been recently discovered in the deepest part of Amazon jungle. So he wrote that these lingam were deposited by the sages who were capable of undertaking astral travel to spread the Message about God to the whole world.

Yog-Siddha could take their consciousness inwards to the tiniest particle in human Being and gain a precise knowledge about Human Anatomy and Physiology [Laghuma]. Or they could expand the consciousness into the cosmos [Mahima] and know precisely about the moments of planets [Astrology and Astronomy] or they develop a very lucid knowledge about the events in the past, present and the future [Trikaldarshi avastha]. The scriptures call it as Turia state of consciousness.

Eight limbed yog of sage Patanjali 2500 years ago promised the conquest of graying of hair, dim vision by cataract, of ageing and diseases by a regular practice of Kriya yog. Shri Ramdeo Baba is an excellent living example of this ancient truth. Today health really means wealth as ill health means financial devastation by costly investigations, expensive interventions and wrong diagnosis.

Kriya is also known as Indian Integral Yog [I.I.Y.]. The short form I I why is the essence of spiritual wisdom. Indian doctors must reduce their I-ness and My-ness in order to undergo transformation of Macaulay programmed rigid mindset [Vrutti]. Even today Indian doctors refuse to accept the ancient Indian art and science of healing and firmly believe that whatever is British or foreign is good and better than our own. Kriya yog depends on Vrutti nirodh for self-transformation

Today, in Iron Age, the Devil or negativity of the mind is most powerful. It destroys a human being in a fraction of a second. Lust is the most powerful weapon of the devil. So in a moment of weakness those who were worshipped became locked in the prison. The soul, mind and body have become weak. It cannot resist falling into "Money trap" or "Honey trap". Politicians, cricketers and even a physician may fall in these two major traps set up by devil. The controlling and ruling power over the agile mind is absent. BK-Rajayoga gives enhancement of power of mind within three months of regular practice. The adherence to moral and ethical values then becomes a second nature and becomes easy and automatic. Stress associated diseases, the NCDs, and addictions are rampant because of the lack of control over mind. Empowered mind cures the diseases as well as brings effective and long lasting De-addiction.

International Yog day is now celebrated all over the world on 21 st of June every year. But in India, the land of spiritual wisdom, anything spiritual becomes the target of vehement controversies. I have submitted a compact and add-on syllabus of mere five lectures and five practical experiential sessions to be conducted only in the first academic term of First to Final M.B.B.S in 2013. Even today it remains in the waste paper basket. Top level medical administrators and policy makers like Vice Chancellors of medical University and MCI refuse to understand that alarming rise in the NCDs like Diabetes, Heart disease, Depression and cancer could not be controlled until man learns to control his agile mind. The maxim "Mind control is the best form of control" adores each and every state transport. But the Indian doctors refuse to believe in this ancient spiritual wisdom. Directorate of Health Services of Maharashtra opened an independent wing of NCD and addictions in the year 2012. But thousands and thousands spent on expensive workshops; mindless workshops have not brought the rise in NCDs under control. Cancer has shown 45 percent rise in India. Child obesity and Attention Deficiency Hyperactive Disease [ADHD] have become a grave problem in adulthood. India has one person in three who is affected by Diabetes and High Blood pressure. Research has shown that mindfulness meditation is the best form of therapy in ADHD. It is gladly accepted by both the parents as well as the patient as an alternative to drugs.

God created a miracle of coronary artery disease regression [CAD-regression] in 2011 by BK-Rajayoga. President Abdul Kalam initiated Mount Abu open Heart Trial in 1998.Sir J J Hospital, Mumbai and Cardiovascular disease Division of University of Alabama, USA were amongst the participants in this multi-centric study conducted by BK Dr. Satish Gupta. A hundred percent disappearance of coronary vessel blocks was obtained in majority of the patients. Another mindboggling miracle was that a phenomenal rise of ejection factor from a base 40 percent to 65 percent was recorded because of the rapid development of collateral circulation. Best efforts by Dr. Navin C. Nanda, USA, could not get this work published in American Heat Journal. After all, India is the million dollar market for the stents. Greed oriented health commerce just could not bear that the Indians shall get rid of heart disease by a regular practice of asana, Pranayam and Meditation. At last it was published in Indian Heart Journal in 2011[63:461-469:2011] after several eminent cardiologists from India attended the famous "Dilwale conference at Mount Abu." This conference had neither alcohol nor non-vegetarian food on agenda and it was totally sponsored by the disease regressed cardiac patients.

Indian doctors must realize that the yog is an ultimate prescription for health, happiness, harmony, peace and prosperity in life. Health is wealth is more pertinent today. Families after families get financially devastated because of expensive investigations and interventions. Common man just cannot afford to fall ill.

A limited unpublished study in the Geriatric OPD of Sir J J Hospital, Mumbai has shown that BK-Rajayoga gives great solace to the troubled aged minds that perpetually dwell upon falling life force energy, stress, financial depletion and severe constipation. Pranayam Motivated Defecation [PMD] gave emancipation from severe constipation.

Practitioners of mainstream medicine must leave aside their personal mind block against Yog and should start experimenting with themselves. Their "Experiences of yog" shall provide "Experiential evidence" for the self. If this happens, then a day shall come when the doctors shall prescribe meditation [BK-Rajayoga] three times a day.

A cardiologist in Jalna, Maharashtra, was motivated to use BK Dr. Chandrasekhar's Happiness Index machine. He started telling his patients that he shall reduce the doses prescribed by him if happiness index is normal. The index never used to be normal. He then would direct them to the BK-Centre for a free of cost Foundation course of mere seven days. He would then advice to practice BK-Rajayoga for three months. At the end of this period, the patients who practiced diligently showed a significant rise in Happiness Index. Their doses of the drugs were reduced. Naturally side effects happened only in negligent proportion of the patients who neglected doing regular practice. His clinical practice rose several folds within a short time.

First develop belief and faith by putting BK-Rajayoga for experimenting in daily routine and get self-acquired experience. "My own experience in the matter has shown that the God starts giving positive strokes with ten days which progressively increase in number and strength. The most intractable problem in life just disappears. Incurable diseases not responding to therapy get completely cured. Self experience is the best teacher in life.

Yog means connection of the sukshma sharir or the soul to the Supreme Consciousness or God for drawing divine qualities and powers from Him. The soul and the mind gets gradually empowered with attainment of a higher and elevated level of pure consciousness. Body becomes strengthened and free of disease automatically because of the release of rejuvenating neuro-hormones from the brain. The essence of yog is to have an elevated Vichar [thought], Achar [Karma], Ahar [Satvik vegetarian food providing balanced nutrition], Vihar [exercise] and vyavhar [Behavior]. Yogasanas maintain the suppleness and the tone of the body and thus are different from gymnastic exercises. Yogasanas teach us the art of mindfulness. Gym exercises only give the bulk and the bulge. The voracious consumption of synthetic protein supplements may damage the natural body mechanisms and thus may be harmful in long run. In fact, a meaningful research is necessary in this area.

PATANJALI KRIYA YOG

It could be divided into two components-
1] Hath-yog and
2] Gyan yog or Rajayog

Hath-yog has four components – Yama, Niyama, Asana and Pranayam.

Gyan yog also has four components – Dhyan, Dharana, Pratyahar and Samadhi [Kaivalya]

All the kriyas must be done with **Ishwer pranidhan** which means a total trusting surrender of the self to God. Adherence to an unshakable single minded spiritual effort [Purusharth] prevent various obstacles and doubts that arise in the mind. BK-concepts call this single-mindedness as **Eknamy is economy.**

Three types of obstacles may arise in spiritual effort-
1. Physical- actual disease of the body and laziness. BK-concepts call it Alasya
2. Mental- Doubts, ego, carelessness, and seeking sexual and sensual gratification.
3. Transcendental- living in a state of hallucination [Bhrum] or may be using hallucinogens or psychedelic drugs like LSD.

STEPS IN HATH-YOG
A] YAMA
1] Yama means restraint or **yoganushasan** under divine guidance or Shrimat.

Five Yamas are Ahinsa – non-violence even in thoughts, Satya or truthfulness even in thoughts, asteya means no-stealing even in thoughts, Brahmacharya means celibacy not only at physical level but even in thoughts and Aparigrah- freedom from greed and avarice.

In short Yamas are powerful Universal vows not be broken under any circumstances.

EFFECTS OF OBSERVING YAMA-

If sadhak adheres to Ahinsa in thoughts and actions then all the living Beings around him abandon the hostile behavior. Remember the pictures of yogi in sadhana surrounded by comfortably lolling tigers and lions and you may realize that thoughts of ahinsa could calm down even the most violent creatures. This technique in BK-Rajayoga involves always having Shubh chintan and Shubh kamana for each and every living being.

Observance of Satya or truthfulness results in spoken words getting translated into reality [Vacha siddhi]. Observance of asteya by sadhak results in getting different kinds of treasures bestowed upon him. The physical celibacy coupled with pure thoughts devoid of lust confers wit, vitality, vigor, unbound energy and spiritual knowledge that flows like a river. Observance of Aparigrah makes sadhak the knower of his past and future in precise terms.

B] NIYAMA

Five Niyamas are Shauch [cleanliness], santosh [contentment], Tapas [Intense meditation or spiritual practice], swadhyaya [study of sacred scripture and that of self] and Ishwer-praniadhan [Total Trusting surrender of self to the God with Vacha, karmana and mana].

Shauch is of two types- External and internal. Daily bathing is external Shauch. Cleansing one's thoughts to the highest grade of purity is known as internal Shauch. Regular [akhandeet] practice of Yama and Niyama helps to achieve Samadhi which means eradication of all the causes of pain, afflictions, diseases and suffering.

YOGASANA AND ITS EFFECTS ON MIND AND BODY

ASANA means positioning the body as a whole with dedication. Spend few seconds in observing the "Experiences" that arise from the pose. When a seeker is closer to a soul conscious state by regular abhayas [practice] of a mindfulness meditation, asana automatically achieves an extension, repose and poise. Effortful effort becomes effortless yogic posture. A combination of effort, concentration and balance in asana automatically forces us to dwell on the present moment. Practice of yogasana must be combined with regular schedule of a mindfulness meditation like BK-Rajayoga. Mindfulness has both strengthening and cleansing effects. At subtlest level achieved by meditation a seeker is able to observe workings of Rajas, Tamas and Sattva in own consciousness. Asana then acts as a bridge that connects body with mind. Seeker fully realizes that his finite body has merged into infinite or the soul. This is perfect yogasana.

C] PRANAYAM

Definition-

Prana means Life force energy. Ayama means ascension, expansion and extension. Pranayam is the expansion of the life force energy through control of the breath.

According to Sankhya philosophy man is composed of five elements-earth, water, air, fire and Aether. Spine is an element of earth. It acts a field for respiration. Distribution and creation of the space in the torso is the function of Aether. Respiration represents the element of air. Remaining two elements water and fire by nature are opposed to each other. The practice of Pranayam fuses them to produce Bio-energy or Life Force energy or Prana.

Pranayam has three components-

1. Inhalation [Poorak]
2. Exhalation [Rechak] and
3. Retention [Kumbhak]. Two types of Kumbhak are Bahya Kumbhak and antar-kumbhak.

Practice of Pranayam removes the veil of ignorance covering the light of intelligence and makes the mind a fit instrument to embark on meditation for the vision of the soul. Pranayam brings such control that it creates an ease in inflow and outflow of the breath. Normal breath flow is irregular. It depends on the emotional state and environment of the person.

TYPES OF PRANAYAM

1] Anulom-vilom or Nadi shuddhi pranayam

2] Kapal bhati

3] Bhasrika

4] Bramari

5] Agnisar

6] Uddiyan bandh

7] Ujjayee

COOLING PRANAYAM

8] Shitali

9] Shitkari

Regular practice of Pranayam modifies inflatory and deflatory lung reflexes. The interaction with central neural elements brings about a new homeostasis or internal balance in the body.

D] PRATYAHARA

This is the next stage in spiritual evolution that one achieves through practice of Yama, Niyama, asana and pranayam. In this stage a seeker achieves the conquest of his senses and mind. The practice of mindfulness meditation enhances achieving this conquest. Senses become quiet and craving for gratification becomes over. Thus the mind attached to senses becomes free [Bandh-mukta] to contemplate over the soul and begins to enjoy new spiritual heights [Atindriya sukh]. All the koshas of the body get purified. An inner bliss ensues.

E] SAMADHI OR KAIVALYA

This term is often confused with suspended animation or Nirvana which is final emancipation from death.. In simplest terms Samadhi means liberation for pain, suffering and diseases.

Sage Patanjali describes eight levels of Samadhi. At what level one becomes a yog-Siddha meaning yogi with super human powers is unknown to me.

The seventh stage is called as Viram Pratyaya or silencing the turbulence of consciousness.[Nirvikar avastha]. The eighth one is known as Nirbeej Samadhi. BK-concepts call this stage as ashariri avyakta avastha or Bindoo roop avastha.

Four initial stages of Samadhi are as follows-

1. Self-analysis.[Swadhyaya] Modern Management Gurus call it as S.W.O.T. analysis.
2. Synthesis [Contemplation, Manan-chintan]
3. State of Bliss [Sat-chit-anand avastha]
4. Experience of pure Being or soul [Soul-conscious state]

The intermediate of fifth and sixth states rapidly progress to elevated seventh and eight stages. Fifth stage is Vikara means assailment by doubts and sixth stage is Vitarka means differentiating the knowledge gained. These two stages indicate a growing body of "spiritual Experience". Gradually developing mental depth makes the pure consciousness to dwell upon self alone. A self realization happens.

In the whole process the movements of consciousness may be cognizable or non-cognizable, painful or non-painful. Pain may be hidden in non-painful state and the non-painful may be hidden in painful state. Thus consciousness perceives the objects according to its own idiosyncrasies and creates fluctuations in one's thoughts. The resultant thoughts when associated with pain or anguish are known as Klesha or a painful state of mind. Pleasing state of mind which exists side by side and which is one of the inherent qualities of the soul is forgotten.

Cognizable pains could be annihilated by practice of yog which enhances will power. In non-cognizable or hidden pains are prevented from arising to the state of cognition by freedom from desires [Nirapeksha avastha]. This is quite important. It has been shown that the cancer patients in terminal stages show a remarkable hardiness to pain if they have been doing some meditative or yogic practices.

Thus it possible to define yog as attaining a restraint over fluctuations of consciousness [Single mindedness] and attain a deep inner silence. [Antar mauna].

Exact meaning of the term Chitta or consciousness is difficult to convey because it is the subtlest form of cosmic intelligence. This is a inner guiding beam which takes every phenomenon to its full evolution meaning a deity like divine, pure and powerful state of consciousness or to the highest awareness of most refined and pure consciousness. BK-concepts define consciousness simply as a combination of awareness with energy, an intelligent energy of unknown nature.

A QUICK -FIX. YOGIC HEALTH- PROGRAMME FOR E.B.P.
[Extremely Busy Persons]

1. A seeker could finish sadhana in just half an hour.Begin the schedule at 4am preferably. This is Brahma muhurt or Amrit vela. Tahjud ki namaz is also done at 4am. This is the most powerful time window for transcendence and connecting with supreme consciousness.
2. Wash your face and then gargle. Subsequently drink 5-6 glasses of plain water or lukewarm water with a pinch of salt if not having high blood pressure. Shauch shall be easy and automatic.

Pranayam Motivated Defecation [P.M.D.]-

Western style commode is necessary. Do movements of abdomen as in Agnisar for some time. Then comfortably visualize that the faecal bolus at caecal end has detached from the colon wall and moving into ascending colon, subsequently into Transverse and Descending colon and finally into the rectum. Visualize the peristaltic waves pushing the bolus to its termination. Carry out this visualization for some time. Once again practice Agnisar. Large quantity of water drunken before facilitates the outcome. Repeat visualization and Agnisar if necessary. Soon the visualization becomes a reality and the movement of bolus is felt. Once one crosses the initial resistance, the fluid movement of the bolus becomes automatic and easy. This technique is very beneficial as it avoids straining during defecation. Many hernias and piles could be prevented if all the persons who exert a lot during defaecation could practice PMD diligently. A limited observation in the Geriatric persons at Sir J J Hospital, Mumbai has given this conclusion.

3. **Pranayam** Nadi-shuddhi is a basic Pranayam. Left nostril kapalbhati [52 times] - this activates the Chandra nadi, Yin energy, feminine energy. Right nostril kapalbhati [52 times]- This activated surya nadi, Yang energy or Male energy. Finally both nostril kapalbhati is done [108 times]. This brings about coherence between Yin and Yang energies and restores the internal balance.

Repeat this entire process- Left nadi Kapalbhati, Right nadi Kapalbhati and both nostrils or sampoorna Kapalbhati three times in one sitting.

Regular practice of Kapalbhati gives Tejas or Noor [glow] on the face without cosmetics in three months.

4. **Mindfulness Meditation program**- Minimum of 30 minutes must be given. In my experience BK-Rajayoga Meditation is the best. It gives BRR and the zone of Dr. Herbert Benson within few seconds or minutes after a regular practice for three months. The seeker feels very light and blissful.

5. **ASANAs**- Three asana in supine position –1] Pavan muktasana, Right pavan muktasana, Left pavan muktasana, Complete pavan muktasana 2] Sarvangasana and 3] Halasana

Instead of number 2 and 3 one could do leg raising- left, right and both legs, maintaining the posture for some time so that a strain is felt in abdominal muscle.

Four asanas in prone position-
1] Bhujangasan
2] Naukasan
3] Makarasan and
4] Ardha shalabhasana [Left], Ardha shalabhasana [right] and both legs shalabhasana.

Asanas in standing position-
1] Surya namaskar - includes twelve asanas and is the best if there is time crunch.

Sun gazing- Eyes are the only windows for energy from sun and cosmic energy to enter the body right up to occipital lobe. Hence surya namaskar is done while gazing at the morning sun. Using goggles prevents energy from entering into body. A research has proved that DNA of the cells stores this cosmic energy which is received in the form of photon or light energy particles.

SUN GAZING IN USA-Hira Ratan Manik Phenomenon[HRM]

Sir J J Hospital, Mumbai invited tenders for solar energy. Mr. Hira Ratan Manik, a retired IAS officer visited Physiology Department as coincidence. He was 75 years old, well-built and was not having spectacles, a common feature at his age. He was living simply by doing Sun gazing for previous fifteen years. This was unbelievable. He went to USA for his experiments in Sun gazing. When I asked –Why USA? He answered –USA is the only country in the whole word which believes in any crazy hypothesis and is willing to spent millions for research. He was under strict medical supervision. Once his BP became as low as 60 mm of Hg. He firmly denied any medical intervention. Soon BP came to normal. Since then he is surviving only by sun gazing. Dr. Cooley, the surgeon who carried out the first heart transplant is one of the sun-gazers. I asked sceptically- But what about UV light in sun rays damaging the eyes? He said-In India there is no danger. But in foreign countries they have photometers in their wrist watches which guide them to safe zones for sun gazing. Sceptical me again asked- What about rainy season or cloudy weather? He told that one could walk on grass with barefoot and whatever energy derived from limited exposure could be harnessed.

A story about Korean prisoners told by him was quite interesting. The prisons were overflowing. So a novel punishment was given. The culprits were made to stand and gaze at the sun for the whole day for some days. At the end of punishment, several of the prisoners donated their specs which they were wearing for last several years. Sun gazing by a miracle has cured their eyesight.

2] Paschimottasan.- sitting position.

NOTE-

1. A seeker must learn and perform yogasana under the observation and guidance of a trained yoga teacher. This prevents assuming some defective posture or doing yogasana in a wrong way. In both cases, the desired and described benefits may not be obtained. Secondly some injury or harm may come. Some money spent on a yoga teacher is a health investment.

2. It is recommended that the seeker may refer to excellent texts like the Textbook of Physiology by Bijalani, Best and Taylor's physiological basis of medical practice and Yogasanas by Swami Sivananda.

PHYSIOLOGICAL EFFECTS OF YOGA

1] Cardiovascular effects- Yogic practices reduce the heart rate and blood pressure. This could be demonstrated by RespErate, a tiny portable instrument with the Medical wing of Brahma Kumaris.

2] Respiratory effects- Yogic practice reduces the resting respiratory rate as shown by Resp-E-rate. Normal rate is 16-18 per minute. The rate may get reduced to 12 per minute by various biofeed and relaxation techniques. But yogic practices may reduce it to two per minute. Further they increase the vital capacity, timed vital capacity, maximum voluntary respiration, breath holding time, and maximum inspiratory and expiratory pressures.

3] CNS effects- Studies by Professor B.K. Anand and at S-VYASA Swami Vivekananda Yog Anusandhan Sanstha have shown that EEG of the yogis shows a preponderance of alpha brain waves. Several practitioners of BK-Rajayoga who meditated for five years or more have shown delta waves of deep sleep in E.E.G. Furthermore, it was observed that sensory stimuli such as a loud bang, or an ice cold or hot object, which normally block the alpha rhythm, could not do so in yogis doing meditation. This absence of alpha blocking indicates that yogis do not easily get distracted by sensory stimuli while they are meditating. An increase in alpha/delta power and a decrease in beta/alpha power also has been recorded. This decrease in beta/alpha power indicated a more relaxed mind during the wakeful period. Further it was observed that there was a better synchrony or coherence between the right and left brain. This indicates enhanced emotional intelligence and creativity. At the same time a significant increase in cutaneous peripheral vascular resistance observed. This indicates a relaxed and alert mind with increased mental alertness.

An increase in Galvanic Skin Response [GSR] or Electro Dermal Response [EDR] indicates a predominance of sympathetic activity. An alerting stimulus eg sudden loud sound leads to palmer sweating. Sweat being a good conductor to fall in the electrical skin resistance. The response is within seconds of stimulus and over within half a minute. The magnitude of response is considered as an indicator of sympathetic activity. Yogis have fewer GSRs than non-meditating controls.

Dr. Herbert Benson- described BRR and the zone in deep meditative states. BRR or Biological Relaxation Response indicates a total physical relaxation. The zone indicates a totally focused and alert mind which also relaxed totally.

Yogis showed better Critical Fusion Frequency [CFF]. This indicates a better neural performance and reduced fatigue and stress level.

Endocrine and Metabolic effects-

Yogic practices have been shown to reduce baseline and average glucicorticoid levels. Similarly they reduce fasting sugar levels and serum cholesterol levels. These indicators suggest a lower risk of Diabetes and Atherosclerosis. Plasma melatonin level was found to be higher. This is one of the factors producing health promoting effect.

MECHANISMS UNDERLYING THE EFFECTS OF YOGA

The mechanisms are not well understood. It is even difficult to determine what may be considered as mechanism. For instance- Higher alpha index in E.E.G. may be considered as a mechanism underlying calm disposition of the yogis. But it may be argued that high alpha index is an effect of yogic practices. Alpha index determination requires a laboratory. Calm disposition could be seen by everybody.

Sometimes some "Mechanisms" or findings search for an effect. For instance- Positron Emission Tomography [PET] in yoga nidra or the deepest meditative state increases cerebral blood flow in sensory and association corticises in the posterior part of the brain. In contrast, in normal resting state, there is high cerebral blood flow in the frontal lobe, basal ganglia, thalamus and cerebellum. Whys such a difference known physiology is unable to explain.

Yogasana increase the strength and efficiency of the muscles and improve the flexibility of the body. This is similar to other exercises. But improvement in cardio-respiratory function seems to be out of proportion to the intensity of yogic exercises in terms of energy expenditure which remains low.

A shift in the autonomic balance towards parasympathetic dominance may explain the reduction in heart rate, fall in blood pressure and improvement in gastrointestinal function.

The increased glucocorticoid secretion in response to an acute challenge may explain the improved ability to cope up with stress.

The physical exercise, dietary changes and stress reduction associated with yogic practices may explain the fall in fasting plasma glucose levels and serum cholesterol levels.

YOGA AS TREATMENT

Yoga has become incorporated in modern medicine in last few decades. There are three reasons for this development-

1] Modern lifestyle diseases like obesity, Hypertension, Diabetes, and heart attacks are on the rise because of the faulty lifestyle. Yoga is the best lifestyle management known to man.

2] Stress is a major killer today. Yoga provides a new way of looking towards life. Hence everything remaining the same, the person starts feeling better [wellness]. This method of changing the perceptive and perception even under changing circumstances is almost infallible. The dictum is face it, fight it and finish it.

3] Emergence of psychoneuroimmunology [PNI] has provided a solid foundation for Mind Body relationship. Science demands scientific evidence. Experiential evidence has no meaning for modern medicine. PNI has acted as a bridge between ancient wisdom and modern medicine. The evidence generated by PNI has made modern medicine accept relaxation, peace, love, hope, happiness and joy as therapeutic tools. Yoga promotes feelings of wellness. Thus concepts of wellness and whole person medicine have arisen in scientific medicine. Not only a cure but the Quality Of Life [Q.O.L.] and Energy, enthusiasm and happiness in life [EEH value] have acquired importance in Healthcare.

Mind Body Medicine has now become the latest frontier in modern medicine and yoga is a potent instrument for influencing the mind positively.

1] Orthopedic problems- Yogasanas have been used for cervical spondylitits and back ache. Benefits accrued from strengthening specific group of muscles. Asanas for relaxation have been used for conditions requiring relief from muscle spasm. A majority of physiotherapeutic measures are usually modified forms of yogasana.

2] Hypertension- Meditation has been shown to reduce systolic and diastolic pressure of hypertensive patients in several studies.

3] Diabetes Mellitus- Dhanurasana was found to be the most effective for Diabetes [Sahay B.K. 1986]. There are some other studies that show improved glycaemic control in Diabetes.

4] Asthma- S-VYASA at Bangalore carried out a large series and proved that selected yogic practices and pranayama reduce the frequency and severity of asthmatic attacks, reduce the requirement of drugs and increases the peak expiratory flow rate.

5] Coronary Artery Disease- Dean Ornish study in 1990 was the beginning. Dr. Satish Gupta [Mount Abu}, Navin C. Nanda [Director of Cardiovascular Division of University of Alabama, USA] and Dr. V. D. Chavan

[Cardiology Division, Sir J J Hospital, Mumbai] carried out Mount Abu Open Heart Trial in 2011 and demonstrated cent percent disappearance of blocks and amazing rise in ejection factor from mere 40% to 65% in just three months.

6] Psychological disorders-

Yogic practices especially meditation has been used professionally for stress reduction in psychiatric disorders. Yogic practices generate happiness and peace. It gives a better insight into the problem and uses the knowledge for recovery just like any other form of counseling. But yogic approach differs in the following way-

Control acquired by the patient is not by trying to change the circumstances and others. This is ego driven approach trying to control others. It has a very limited scope. Patient tries to change his perception and his way of looking at the circumstances and the persons. Thus it is the principle of self-transformation for world transformation. BK-Mediation gives the best results in self-transformation. In modern psychology it is known as cognitive re-appraisal.

7] Cancer-Psycho-oncology – Mindfulness program or meditation harnesses the immense healing power of the mind. Several have become cancer free in Carl Simonton study and Bernie Siegel follow up.

Meditation, Types, Mindfulness, Inner Silence, Focus, SWOT Analysis and Out of Box Thinking

Definition of Meditation.

There is an urgent need for bringing out a **universally accepted and lucid definition** of the ancient Indian complex process of Meditation that brings about healing of the self, and then progresses to self-realization and achievement of the final goal of this spiritual and yogic practice.

Author proposes that the following may be considered as candidates for a **flawless definition** of meditation for universal acceptance-

Meditation is a complex ancient Indian yogic practice **[Sadhana]** inherently having two components- Dhyan and Dharana which transforms the basal Rajasik-Tamasik consciousness to higher or elevated powerful and pure Satvik consciousness or soul consciousness giving the forgetfulness of the mundane terrestrial and transient bonds of the material world because of a transcendence of consciousness. Obtaining Peace, love, happiness, harmony, **health** and prosperity become an easy and automatic achievement. Transcendence is limitless and the human being could acquire **super human powers** like sankalpa siddhi, vacha siddhi, levitation, walking on fire or water, clairvoyance; travel in cosmos in astral form, kaya kalpa and par-kaya pravesh or suspended animation. Most important is that the meditation practice must give the ability called **mindfulness**. The person must acquire **controlling and ruling powers over mind** so that he shall be able focus on a particular positive thought in moment without any time lapse for any length of time.

WHY PRECISE AND UNIVERSALLY ACCEPTED DEFINITION IS NECESSARY?

1] Meditation research all over the world suffers as mere relaxation procedures are also considered as meditation which is wrong. So whatever one research considers as best may not be the best at all.

2] Indian Integral yog or Ashtang yog or Kriya yog of sage Patanjali has eight components or practices [Kriya] for **conquest over ageing and diseases**. Dhyan and Dharana are the two components which form the complete and complex process of meditation.

3] As the **gold standard is absent** in definition, the results of different forms of meditation cannot be compared for determining the best procedure or technique.

4] Final goal of performing the complex procedure of **acquiring transcendence** is not defined in any of the studies. Hence anything and everything could be made to appear good and better than the others.

5] Same form of meditation technique has acquired different names- for instance-

Vipassana is the original Buddhist form of meditation as told to humanity by Lord Gautama Buddha and it is the original and true Art of living. Today several variations of the same basic technique have become very famous – for instance –

Art of Living by Sri Sri Ravishankar, Preksha Dhyan of **Jainism**, Japanese Zen Meditation, Chinese **Tai chi**, Korean meditation, Tibetan meditation of Lamas.

Transcendental Meditation [TM] of Maharshi Mahesh yogi became most popular and was subjected to extensive research because Maharshi performed act of levitation that is- walking over fire or water in USA.

More recently Sri Sri Ravishankarji's **Sudershan Kriya** which is now commercially available at a cost of few thousands has become a status symbol. It has become a current fashion and craze.
No wonder the scriptures describe kali yug or Iron Age as an era of gross mental confusion [Bhrushta **mati**].

6] Precise knowledge about certain metaphysical entities and phenomena is necessary to understand **the complex process of ancient Indian meditation**. For instance- soul, God, consciousness, energy chakra, body aura, soul as transmitter of thought vibrations, Life

Force energy and several others. Such knowledge is absent in most of the research publications. Consciousness remains an enigma even today to the topmost scientists in the field of Artificial Intelligence [AI]. Exactly for this reason they have not been able to introduce Emotional Intelligence in robots. Life Force energy **[Prana]** is an unknown form of vibrational energy which again is an enigma for the scientists. The concept of **"Specific Energy Signature"** in the tissue getting damaged or diseased by trauma or pollution and translating into ailments is new. The concept of flow of cosmic energy into body through **Cosmic Healing Vibrational whisper** by meditation and enhancing soul and mind power is also not universally accepted for the lack of scientific evidence. However **"experiential evidence"** about the same is universal in yogic practitioners. Same could be told about the "Experience" of mental peace and mental empowerment after meditation.

7] **Scientism**- This is a modern mental affliction which demands scientific proof before having **belief and faith** which are most essential for a yogic practice. The term total trusting surrender has been used by sage Patanjali. In recent times several studies have appeared in which placebos or non-medicinal substances become 70 to 300 times more potent than the drugs if the person has belief and faith in the treating physician.

8] Spiritual and yogic knowledge has been derived from the "Mystical Experiences" **[Sakshatkar]** to highly evolved and enlightened souls. But the medical science dismisses mystical experiences as hallucinations [Bhrum] as both phenomena occur in the same area of the cortex.

9] The following instruments are with BK-R.E.R.F. – Rajayoga Education and Research Foundation [Medical wing] which demonstrate the deep meditative "Experiences". But they **require scientific validation-**
Thought graph machine, Aura scanner, RespErate, Portable aura scanner [modified Universal scanner] and Happiness Index Machine.

10] US National Centre of Complementary and Alternative Medicine [NCCAM] in 2005 defined meditation as conscious mental process that induces a set of physiological changes termed as Biological Relaxation Response **[B.R.R.].** This definition is largely responsible for confusion that perceives meditation as a simple relaxation technique.

11] US NCCAM in 2006 gave a revised definition-
Meditation is a process in which the person learns to focus his attention on a single positive thought or a Point and to suspend the stream of thoughts which are often negative and which usually occupy his mind. This practice results in great physical relaxation, mental calmness and psychological balance.

12] In several publications US NCCAM 2006 is not mentioned. Instead a variety of terms like Sahaj Rajayoga [of Nirmala Devi], or Brahma kumaris Rajayoga or Swami Shivanand/ Nityanand- Math or Tibetan meditation are mentioned. The details of technique are never available. This becomes a hurdle in scientific comparison. Globally such techniques shall never be accepted because of the religious bias. A scientific definition shall remove such objections.

13] Dr. Richard Davidson, Professor of Psychiatry, Wisconsin University, and USA coined a term Mindfulness Meditation which denotes inclusion of Dhyan and Dharana though not specified so clearly.

ANCIENT INDIAN DEFINITION OF MEDITATION [SAGE PATANJALI]

Meditation is a complex technique consisting **of Dhyan and Dharana** performed with aim of spiritual evolution leading to transformation of one's Nature **[Vrutti]** from basal Tamasik/Rajasik consciousness to higher and powerful **Satvik or soul consciousness** to the highest level called as **Turia consciousness** [Trikaal-darshi] through **eight levels** of Samadhi or Kaivalya by vrutti-nirodh and ishwer-pranidhan. Conquests over graying of hair, dim vision, ageing and diseases are incidental benefits. Vrutti nirodh means gradual diversion of desires and negative thoughts and emotions for getting control over mind. Ishwer-praniadhan means a total

214

trusting surrender to God. A sadhak must learn to focus on the thoughtless interval happening between two thoughts and learn to increase this interval by regular Sadhana or meditative practice. Trikaal-darshi means the knowledge of past and future becomes known in very precise terms.

This component of **thoughtless interval** introduces a novel concept of **Non-thought consciousness.** Author personally has tried to achieve this state but failed for nearly three years of practice of Kriya yog. **BK-Rajayoga made everything easy, quick and automatic.** Mind is agile like a monkey which has been bitten by thousand scorpions. Main function of the mind is to have thoughts, emotions and desires. Author believes that only the dead in the grave could have Non-thought consciousness. A thoughtless situation means vacuum in the mind. Nature always tries to fill the vacuum. **In BK- Rajayoga purging of negativity is associated with concomitant re-writing the corrupted CD of the mind by positive thoughts.** Once positive thoughts become entrenched deep in psyche by autosuggestion and visualization, Satvik consciousness becomes a second nature. Then the perception, attitude and behavioral pattern become elevated and uncontaminated with desires of self-gain, negative thoughts or emotions. **Strict adherence to moral and ethical values becomes automatic and easy.**

Note- This is the most simplified version of the definition given by yog-shreshtha BKS Iyengar.

TYPES OF MEDITATIONS

Presently meditation techniques could be classified into two categories-
1] Concentrative forms or relaxation oriented meditations
2] Mindfulness type or Inner silence oriented meditations.
Dr. Richard Davidson, Professor of Psychiatry, Wisconsin University, USA, coined the term Mindfulness Meditation. In recent times, various Mindfulness based programs have been used for stress management, mind empowerment and cancer cure.

CONCENTRATIVE TYPE

All of these are relaxation oriented meditations. So they do not fit into a complete definition of ancient Kriya yog.

For instance- repeated chanting of Kalama, Mantra or God's name is concentrative form of meditation. Transformation of nature [Vrutti] may happen slowly or it may not happen at all in this Iron Age when the mind is weak and lacks self-determination, self-dedication and self-discipline. The person is unable to carry forth regular Sadhana as apart of his daily routine because of laziness and carelessness. **BK- Rajayoga** calls this **alasya**

and albelapan as the two most powerful and subtle or micro forms of attack from Maya or Devil which **makes the person to leave the God's path and the spiritual practice.**

MINDFULNESS MEDITATION

An active and conscious meditation that confers the ability for mindfulness which means a ruling and controlling power over the agile mind to get it focused on the present moment. Eventually a transformation of nature to positivity happens.

Every moment is important because a moment before it was one's future and a moment later it becomes one's past. So if one can take to make the present moment full of health and happiness then one can be sure that the whole life shall be spent in health and happiness.

Following are evidence based Mindfulness Meditations-
1] Zen Meditation
2] Maharshi Mahesh Yogi's Transcendental meditation,
3] Vipassana
4] Brahma Kumaris Rajayoga
5] Preksha Dhyan of Jainism and
6] Art of Living [A.O.L.] by Sri Sri Ravishankerji.

BK-RAJAYOGA

Preamble-

Brahma Kumaris is a N.G.O. that has global presence with more than 11500 Yog-centers in 140 countries. This selfless N.G.O. has won six international peace awards and has **consultative status in U.N.O.** Dadi Janaki; the international Head of the organization has been certified as the **most stable mind** in the whole world by two independent American and Australian groups of Neurophysiologists. Thus she could be the living example of **sthit-pragnya state** of consciousness described in Bhagavad Gita. **The spiritual version of meditation** is taught free of cost in all the centers in a seven days' Foundation course. Thus if BK-Rajayoga becomes accepted by the Healthcare Profession as **evidence based approach to maintenance of health,** then it could become a **global strategy** for health and shall make the celebration of International Yog Day more meaningful. The W.H.O. slogan of **"Health for all"** given in year 2000 may soon become a reality.

Unique Features of BK-Rajayoga

1] It is an inner silence oriented meditation.

2] Easy three step meditation for Extremely Busy Persons- Focus, Internalization and Cosmic communion.[This may mean the vaman avatar in scriptures].

Vipassana has four steps. There is no concept of God or supreme power. Preksha Dhyan has seven steps and it is a variation of Vipassana.

3] Easy definition and easy to understand and practice.
Yog means establishing the connection between the soul, a conscient, metaphysical point of light in the center of the forehead and Supreme soul, Who is also a conscient point of light and drawing powers from the Supreme Powerhouse. This empowerment is the **Dhyan** component. Once soul or mind is empowered then **Dharana of divine values and virtues** or inculcating values as an inseparable part of one's psyche becomes automatic and easy.

4] Release of rejuvenating neurohormones making the conquest of graying, dim vision, ageing and diseases become a reality.

5] Once a person accepts Rajayoga as an integral part of his daily routine, **de-addiction remains permanent and lifelong.**

6] Internal silence of the dominant scientist mind brings the immense potential and wisdom of the Spiritualist mind or subconscious mind into action. Once this happens, impossible becomes I am Possible. Stress management happens by self-management leadership [SML]. An Out Of Box thinking or Lateral thinking by spiritualist mind begins. Linear judgmental thinking by scientist mind stops.

An atman to atman transpersonal human transaction begins. This helps to deal with other person as **soul-brother** with equal potential and wisdom. So relationships in life, marriage, love and at work place improve tremendously.

Instant two seconds judgments become most accurate decisions in life.

Creativity innovation happens in art, scientific research and in problem solving.

7] Waste or negative thinking is the **greatest psychic energy vampire**. It weakens the soul and mind. Futile and useless contemplation [manan-chintan] by **turbulent scientist mind** stops. All the queue of questions, doubts and diseases disappear with surprising ease. An unexplained and unlimited inner tranquility and happiness ensues.

8] Neuro-Linguistic Programming [N.L.P.] to create a Passion Quotient becomes easy.
Note- Thus BK-Rajayoga helps to excel in IQ – Intelligence Quotient [by neurogenesis by BDNF], Passion Quotient [P.Q.], S.W.O.T. analysis, Happiness Quotient [HQ], Moral Quotient [MQ], Emotional Intelligence [EQ] and Spiritual Quotient [SQ].

Improved SQ gives emancipation from Spiritual Vacuum, a term coined by Dr. N.N. Wig, Professor Emeritus of Psychiatry, PGI, and Chandigarh.

SOME EXAMPLES OF WASTE CONTEMPLATION

Turbulent scientist mind raised following several questions amongst which following were most common - Today I conclude that they were the result of **my ego driven intellect.**

1] Past Life Regression hypnosis and therapy has proved the concept in Bhagavad Gita that a single soul takes several births in several different bodies. Kaundinya was the first and foremost amongst the five disciples of Lord Gautama Buddha- Vappa, Bhadheya, Mahanam and Ashwajeet. Was I that evolved and enlightened Kaundinya in previous birth?
Completion of the part of bhakti Yog leads to Gyan Yog or Rajayoga. So is it that my Bhakti yog was completed as Gautama Buddha or Jesus Christ or any one such spiritually evolved and enlightened person?

2] God is omnipresent. So is it not a sin to walk on earth or floor where God is present?

3] God is ageless and deathless or Ajanma. So how Lord Ram or Lord Krishna or God in any body form could be the Supreme Soul or Param Atma ?

4] All human beings believe that God is one. Or how could Rama and Krishna both could be a God? How one could explain thirty three crores of Gods and Goddesses in Hindu religion? Secondly a large number of human beings in the world do not perceive Krishna or Rama as their God. So how any one of them could fulfil the criteria for becoming God in Whom whole of humanity could have have faith as their God?

5] Other religions do not have Goddesses. They have God and angels. Does it mean that the women folk in those religions could never attain a Goddess like status?

6] One more question always plagued me- Who came first on earth, Rama or Krishna? Why chanting always has both the names? This state of affairs is called as **Vyabhichari Bhakti** or worshipping multiple Gods according to BK-concepts as told by incorporeal God through a human conduit.

7] All other religions believe that God is Light. So how come Hindu religion has body forms of thirty three crores of Gods and Goddesses ?

8] Who is Supreme Godhead in ISKON?
BK-Rajayoga gave the most logical and scientific explanations. So contentment came. The Self started singing – Paana thaa so paa liya, ab kuch baki na raha meaning **whatever has to be obtained I have gained**. So nothing remains to be gained.

9] Waste thoughts and negative thinking used to give tiredness. Fatigue disappeared rapidly. Sleep became deep and rejuvenating. Diseases disappeared. A quantum jump in the quality of life [QOL] ensued. Energy, Enthusiasm and Happiness [EEH value] in life increased phenomenally for others to see and tell.

Novel Instruments With R.E.R.F. [BK-Medical Wing] And BK-S.P.A.R.C. Wing For Demonstrating Deep Meditative Experiences

PREAMBLE-

Rajayoga Education and Research Foundation of Brahma Kumaris have several wings like Medical wing and S.P.A.R.C. wing [Spiritual Advancement Research Center].

Spiritual Knowledge is the conglomerate of knowledge derived from "Experiences" and "Mystical Experiences" given by an **incorporeal God** to spiritually evolved and enlightened souls. **Holy Quran** took birth through mystical experiences to **Messiah, Mohammad Paigamber**, the last and the greatest amongst God's Messengers. But present times are such that Devil or Shaitan is luring away the God's children from **Sirat al mustaqim** or Straight Path at alarming speed. It looks as if the Devil shall win the challenge he has given to **The One and Only One, All Merciful Allah**. So in all probability, The Supreme took mercy on His beloved children and sent an additional Messiah, **Brahma Baba** who was a Diamond merchant in Karachi, Pakistan. This development gives a new meaning to the word-Pakistan- meaning a **land of purity**.

"Experiences" and "Mystical Experiences" could not be demonstrated by the help of scientific instruments. As yet no scientific instrument has been able to demonstrate the **sweetness** in the sugar. But this does not mean that sweetness does not exist. This simple logic does not carry far with **Scientist Minds and with the doctors in India**. They demand scientific proof for the existence of soul, God and transcendental experiences by deep meditative practice. **Experiential evidence** actually is enough proof. Millions believe in God on the basis of "Experiential evidence."

Medical wing and S.P.A.R.C. wing have certain novel instruments to show a demonstrable effect of deep meditative experiences. Mystical experiences [Sakshatkar] and Hallucinations [Bhrum] occur in the **same area of cerebral cortex or brain**. Science the infant has not been able to develop a device that could differentiate between **Bhrum and Sakshatkar.**

The next problem with the instruments with medical and S.P.A.R.C. wings is that they need to be validated by medical research institutes by well-planned studies.

There are hardly any scientific ways by which deep meditative experiences could be translated into scientific evidence except for a state of art chemiluminiscence machine that exists in the Biochemistry Department of Sir J J Hospital, Mumbai. It is in use for demonstrating the release of rejuvenating neuro-hormones during BK-Rajayoga Mindfulness meditation. One research project has already been completed. These neurohormones are as under-

1] The rejuvenating neurohormones and the stress relief markers are as under – Serotonin, GABA, DHEA [Dihydro-epi- andosteron] Endorphin, melatonin, cortisol as stress marker and an enzyme called acetyl choline esterase. In addition rejuvenating neuro-hormones like Encephalin, Melatonin, Sirtuins, Brain Derived Neuro-trophic Factor **[BDNF]**, Receptor Modulation Factor **[RMF]** and Stem Cell Activation Factor **[SCAF]** could be estimated. Advanced **chemiluminiscence machine** at Sir J J Hospital could rapidly estimate these markers along with routine blood estimations like blood sugar, urea etc.

2] Use of various Bio-feed back instruments based on demonstration of Galvanic Skin Resistance [GSR].

3] Instruments for demonstrating Heart Rate Variability.

4] Novel Instruments with S.P.A.R.C. and Medical wings of Brahma Kumaris for demonstrating deep meditative experiences -

A] Thought graph machine   B] Kirlian Body Aura scanner   C]Portable aura scanner of BK Dr. Chandrashekhar

D] RespErate machine   E] Happiness Index machine of BK Dr. Chandrashekhar

5] Kirlian Body aura photography with Gas Diffusion Visualization

Change in Body aura is believed to be an earliest sign of onset of a disease. But Padmabhushan Dr. R.D. Lele and several others believe that body aura is an artifact. An open mind is required for carrying out a meaningful research to prove the truth.

DETAILS ABOUT NOVEL INSTRUMENTS

A] Happiness Index machine of BK Dr. Chandrashekhar [Figure-1]
This ingenuous device is again the brainchild of BK Dr. Chandrasekhar and it costs only 1000 Rupees.

Personal Experience-
My lecture on Mind Body Medicine was arranged at IMA Jalna, Maharashtra by my classmate and a renowned Pediatrician Dr. Bhala. One cardiologist purchased the machine under the impact of my lecture. Few years later he phoned me that his practice has now increased manifold because of the use of Happiness Index machine.

He would prescribe drugs after clinical examination. Then he used to tell the patient that if he has normal happiness index then he shall reduce the dosage by half. He soon found that **outwardly happy person may not be internally happy.** Upon this he used to direct the patient to BK-Center of Jalna wherein he was told to practice Rajayoga using the full and proper technique **[Vidhi se hi siddhi hai] for a minimum of three months.** Re-examination after three months, patient who practiced Rajayoga diligently used to show normal happiness index. The attendance **at Jalna center** increased manifolds after these events became common news.

BK-Meditation Hut at Sir J J Hospital, Mumbai under aegis of Ghodapdeo center intended to carry out such meaningful studies. But administrative obstructions are taking their toll.

B] RespErate Machine [Figure -2]

Dr. Naras Bhat [Cardiologist in USA running a Stress clinic] devised this instrument. The electrode could be fitted to a finger by welcro. The small instrument has programmed music which could be listened by two ear plugs and which **gives mental relaxation**. Or otherwise the person could practice his own relaxation technique or meditation and see the computerized reading on a screen. Deeper stages of meditation are indicated by lowering of the rate of respiration. Normal rate is **16 to 18 per minute.** The persons trained in Biofeedback could reduce it to **12 per minute** but not beyond.

Unique personal experience-
Dr. Mrs Kaundinya showed a reduced rate of **7 per minute** by BK-Rajayoga. Both Dr. Bhat and she tested mine. It came to phenomenal and even today **unbelievable 2 per minute** in my case with BK-Rajayoga. Unfortunately I did not purchase the machine costing 300 dollars in 2005. The machine is available with an US company Intereqve, Railey Drug store, California

C] Portable Aura scanner of BK Dr. Chandrasekhar [Figure-3]
The device is actually a universal scanner with two movable electrodes charged with a negative charge. The electrodes move away from each other if there is no barrier between them as the same electric charge repels each other.

On the other hand if there is a barrier of positive energy in between two electrodes, then they remain parallel to each other.

BK Dr. Chandrasekhar shows blocks **in energy chakra** and the size of the body aura by using this instrument.

Unique Personal experience-
I went to Nagpur for a lecture on Mind Body Medicine at NKP Salve Medical Institute of Postgraduate Research. I went for Murali to the BK-centerwhich was nearby where Chandrashekharbhaiji tested my aura.

The size of the aura was significant – **about 90 feet** in length. **Normal aura is 12 feet** and above. But there was a **block in Manipura chakra**. When asked if I have a sensitive GIT, I answered affirmatively. Bhaiji then advised me to increase the dose of **amrit vela meditation.** Since then I started amrit vela from 3.30 am. Six months later, BK-centre at Ghodapdeo invited BK Dr. Chandrasekhar for a talk and demonstration. My aura on this occasion was beyond **135 feet and the block in Manipura chakra had gone.**

D] Kirlian Body Aura scanner [Figure-4]
This expensive machine has been purchased recently when S.P.A.R.C. wing could convince Rameshbhaiji few days before he left the mortal coil.

Dadi Janaki showed a body aura which expanded beyond the recording screen with deepening meditation when tested by Kirlian Body Aura photography with Gas Diffusion Visualization [GDV] technique.

E] Thought Graph Machine [Figure-5]
Several eminent persons like BK Dr. Girish Patel were not aware about the existence of this novel machine.
This machine looks like a computer screen having two keys on which two fingers are kept. A graph shows on the screen. A count below 5000 shows a stress prone personality. Such person is likely to develop one or more stress born **NCDs or Non-infectious Chronic**

Diseases. A count above 10000 shows a stable mind like **Dadi Janaki**. The intermediate counts showed any normal type of personality.

Advanced program shows deep blue water of sea in which a **fish** is swimming. With deepening meditation, the fish develops into a **mermaid** and finally into a **man** eventually. The man starts walking indicating a further deepening. Suddenly a mountain comes in way. If the meditation becomes still deeper, the man develops wings and a sign flashes on the screen- **"Congratulations. You have become an angel."**

Unique personal experience-
When I went to Gyan sarovar, Mount Abu for the first time I was passing through a difficult situation in my life. So mind was stressful. Even then my count came to 14000. So the BK-scientist put me on advanced program. The fish became angel within a few minutes. **Verdict given to me was that I have a stable mind like Dadi Janaki.** On that occasion my mind was stressful and I did not know anything about **Dadi Janaki.** So like a typical person from modern mainstream medicine I **dismissed the verdict as an artifact.**

But once again I got myself tested to prove to my wife Dr. Mrs. Surekha Kaundinya, the value of BK-Rajayoga. I became angel within few minutes. Dr. Surekha struggled for as many as twelve times But the fish never progressed beyond mermaid stage. This was surprising because she has more equipoise than myself and usually very calm under any circumstance. I am more volatile in temper.This incidence was probably a divine plan to convince Mrs Surekha about the power of transformation by BK-Rajayoga.She then started attending Muralis.

Same result on both the occasions-
1] stressful initial phase and
2] five years later made me come to a conclusion.

Thought graph machine probably indicates the basic but definite nature[Vrutti] of a person which he has acquired as Prarabdha [Sanchit karma] of past birth.
This machine appears to be most essential equipment in the studies related to Mind Body Medicine.

Novel Instruments for Demonstrating Deep Meditative Experiences

Happiness Index Machine

RESPeRATE

Portable Aura Scanner

KIRLIAN Body Aura Photograph

BIBLIOGRAPHY

1. Dey NC- Medical Bacteriology. Publisher –Allied Agency, 2-Cornwallis Street, Calcutta-6,2nd Ed. P.-1-9:1962

2. Sheridan JF et al-Psychoneuroimmunology- Stress effects on the pathogenesis and immunity during infection- Clinical Microbiol. Reviewsp.200-212:1994

3. Sharma A. Spirituality and mental health- Reflections of the past, applications in the present and projections of the future.Editor Avadesh Sharma,Publisher Indian Psychiatry Society and R.E.R.F. [Medical Wing] of Brahmakumaris. 5-21,26, 30,32,39,-42,126,:2009

4. Hegde BM-De-schooling medical education. Bhavan's journal.vol54,No24:33-41-July 2008

5. Taimini IK- The science of yoga.The theosophical publishing house. Madras .1961.

6. Marshal Govindan-Babaji and the eighteen Kriya yog siddha tradition. Kali Yog Kriya ashram,Green valley lake,California.1990

7. BKS Iyengar- Light on Yog sutras of Patanjali.Publisher-Harper Collins.p. 133,173,200,233,235,247,252,253 and 255:1993

8. Kinsel JF, Strauss SE- Complementary Alternative therepies.Rigorous research needed

to support claims. Annual Rev. Pharmacol, Toxicol. -43:463:2003

9. Bijlani RL, Manjunatha S.- Understanding Physiolgy- A Text book for medical students. Yoga- Publisher JP Brothers Medical publishers[P] Ltd.,New Delhi India. P.475-773-2011

10. Tandon OP, Tripathy Y.- Best & Taylor's Physiological basis of medical practice.Yoga-Phyasiology and application , therapy and rehabilitation.1217-1230-2012

11. Chinmayanand S- Mandukya Upanishad. Sachin Publishers.Bombay.1984

12. Essen et al- Trends in alternative medicine use in United States. Results of follow up,National Survey wef 1990-1997. JAMA 280:1569:1998

13. Naras Bhat- How to reverse and prevent heart disease and cancer?. Publisher New Editions Publishing,1657, Rollins Roadside B-3,Burlingame,California94010.p.62-103: 1995

14. Benson H, Beary JF, Carol: Relaxation Response. Psychiatry 37:37-46:1974.

15. Gladwell M- Blink- The power of thinking without thinking. Penguin Books. USA 2005

16. Maulana Wahiduddin Khan- The Quran Goodword Books, New Delhi. 2009

17. Kaundinya SD, Kaundinya DV- Meditation versus Relaxation. International J. of Basic & Applied Physiology. Vol. 2[1]:240-257:2013

18. Stancier KM- The Qi Long database – quoted in reference no. 17.

19. Wilcock D. – The source field investigations.The hidden science and lost civilizations behind the 2012 prophecies . Plume publishing.The Penguin group.USA 2011.

20. Patil DD et al –Alchemy of God- Research group for unification of science and spirituality. alchemyofgod108@gmail.com, www.alchemyofgod.com

21. Naras Bhat- Reversing stress and burn out. Cybernatix publishing. California.USA.219-249:2002

22. Gupta Satish et al-Regression of coronary atherosclerosis through healthy lifestyle in coronary disease patients. Mount Abu Open Heart Trial.63 : 461-469 :2011

23. Manocha R et al- Changing definition of meditation.Is there a physiologic corollary?Skin temperature changes of mental silence form of meditation compared to rest.J. of International Society ,Life info.Science. 28[1]:23:2010

24. Davidason R.- Alteration in brain and immune functions produced by Mindfulness Meditation. Psychosomatic medicine.65:564-570 : 2003

25. Shapiro SL, Walsh R, Britton WB- Analysis of recent meditation research and suggestions for future directions. J of Meditation and Meditation Research vol [3],310:57-60-2001

26. Telles Shirley et al al- Heart rate variability spectrum during Vipassana meditation.J Indian Psychology .23:1-5: 2005

27. Kaundinya DV- Rajayoga- evidence based mental silence type of meditation. International J of Current Medicine and Applied Sciences. July 2014

28. Sukhsohale Neelam D et al- Does Rajayoga meditation bring out physiological and psychological general well being amongst the practitioners of it? Internationall J. of Collaborative Research on Internal Medicine and Public health- .vol-4 [no12]: 2000-2009: 2012

29. Telles Shirley, Desiraju T- Autonomic changes in Brahma Kumaris Rajayoga meditation International J Psychophysiology .15: 147-152 :1993

30. Shirley Telles, Navin KV- Changes in middle latency auditory evoke potentials during meditation. Psychophysiological Reports.94:368-400 : 2004

31. Smith WP, Crompton WC, West WB- Meditation as an adjunct to happiness enhancement programme J. Clinical Psychology 51[2] : 269-273 : 1995

32. Wilber K, Walsh R.- An integral approach to consciousness research- A proposal for integrating first, second and third person

approach   to   consciousness.
2002b quoted by ref. 17

33. Reibel DK et al- Mindfulness based Stress Reduction Programme and health related quality of life in heterogeneous patient population in a general hospital. Psychiatry : 23[4]: 2001

34. Carlson LE et al- Mindfulness based Stress Reduction in relations to quality of life ,mood, symptoms of stress, and levels of cortisol, Dihydro-epi-androsteron sulphate [DHEA] and melatonin in breast and prostrate cancer patients. Psycho-neuro-endocrinology : 29[4] :448-474:2004

35. Goleman D-The meditative mind- varieties of meditative experiences.Penguin Putnam,New York.1996.

APPENDIX – I

Total Health Programme [T.H.P.]   <u>Free of Cost</u>
Spiritual Health Clinic
Lecture Hall, St. George Hospital, Near C.S.T., Mumbai

AIMS- [BK-COLABA CENTRE]
1. MY SOCIETY, A HAPPY AND HEALTHY SOCIETY.
2. MY HOSPITAL, ADDICTION FREE HOSPITAL

Components of Total Health Programme [09-01-2015]
1. Current Research in Mind Body Medicine - Dr. Dilip V. Kaundinya MD
2. Sukshma Yogabhyas -
3. Pranayama-
4. Scientific BK-Rajayoga- Mindfulness Based Stress Reduction Programme- [R-MBSRP]-
5. Pranayama Motivated Defecation [P.M.D.] – discussed in Appendix-2.

PREAMBLE-
Warning- All type of **asana** and **Shuddhi Kriya** must be performed under the supervision of a **trained yoga teacher** until one gets proficient.

Diet- Yogic Satvik vegetarian food though not mandatory, is helpful in attaining the higher spiritual levels quickly. One must remember that the journey of the spiritual path is long and there are **eight levels of Samadhi in spiritual elevation** and evolution.

Non-vegetarian diet gives shortening of telomeres and early ageing. A homemade Maharashtrian thali is the most balanced diet amongst various choices available. **Padmabhushan Dr. R.D. Lele** has described various **anti-oxidants and immune modulators** in this vegetarian diet in his wonderful book- Ayurveda and modern medicine, published by **Bharatiya Vidya Bhavan, Mumbai, 2001.**

Garlic and onion in food are Tamasik i.e. they generate laziness and sluggishness of mind. Author has experimented and discovered that the Total Relaxation Response of Mind and Body [Biological Relaxation Response, BRR and the Zone, [Ekagra Chitta avastha] is delayed while meditating when such diet or stale food is ingested. Anything that is not prepared freshly or stored in a refrigerator is considered as stale in Yogism.

2.1] It is **customary but not mandatory** to begin Yogic practices by chanting a Mantra.

A] **Sarve sukhinaha santu, Sarve santu niramaya, Sarve bhadrani paschyantu, - maa pasche dukh makpunyat.**

Let all the divine persons be happy and disease free. Even the lowest of animals may be protected for their welfare. If we do not give pain to others, the pain and suffering shall never come our way.

OR

B] Aum chanting - Laghu Omkar and Dirgh Omkar

OR

C] **Gayatri mantra** may be recited for 11 times with **proper phonetics** [vaikhari], Upanshu [mumbling tones or 3] by silently chanting. Gayatri mantra is a **Beej mantra.** That means though a proper phonetics is essential for maximum benefit, a practitioner **may begin chanting in any way.** Over a period of time Divine Grace **[Insha Allah]** gradually brings an improvement to the proper level of pronunciation. Author has experienced this phenomenon. Gayatri Mantra is said to potentiate power of differentiation between right and wrong or Vivek. [Buddhi shuddhak]. **Buddhi or wisdom is different from intelligence.** Intelligence is an ability to learn the skills of livelihood quickly. Wisdom is the ability of the person to use his God given intellect properly in accordance with the **eternal laws of morals and ethics.**

An unpublished study tells that the **basal life force energy [Prana]** that exists in and around us is at the level of **2-3 photons** [Light energy particles]. With regular chanting the energy levels may raise upto 5 photon units. A human being can never progress to seven or eight photon level or the level of **the 8th Sun.** Aditya is the first Sun.

2.2] **Sukshma Yogabhyas** includes training in some simple yogic postures for protecting your neck, shoulder, lower back, knees and ankles and maintaining them in a resilient state throughout life.. Annamaya Kosh is made free of impurities. Deep abdominal breathing technique, a cyber-scan with Heartfelt Resonant imaging [HRI] is done prior to the Kriya.

1] Calana Kriya- Loosening practices:- This Kriya help to improve micro-circulation.
A] Neck bending, rotation and twisting
B] Kati Shakti vikasak [Trunk movement]
C] Knee movements
D] **Simple yogic postures [Yogasana]** which could be done at any age. Thus this Sukshma Yogabhyas becomes useful for Geriatric patients and could be implemented in various Geriatric O.P.D.s

Eg. **Tadasana, Vakrasana, Ardha chakrasana, Trikonasana, Ardhaustrasana,** [in supine posture]:- Pavan muktasana, Sarvangasana, Halasan and Shavasana **[Relaxing posture]**. These yogic postures are performed in prone posture]:- Bhujangasana, Shalabhasana, Naukasana and Makarasana **[relaxing posture].** Optional- Uttan tadasana and Vishnu shayyasana

2] **Shuddhi Kriya-** Jala neti, Sinha Mudra, Ashwini Mudra [prevents piles and prolapse of rectum] should be done daily
Jal dhoti should be done daily for one month. Later it should be done on every first day and fifteenth day of each month.

Advanced Yogabhyas includes 1] pada hastasana,2] Bhadrasana3] Ardha matsyendrasana,4] Dhunurasana 5]Matsyasana 6]Pachimotanasana and 7] nauli

2.3] **Pranayama-** Eight types of Pranayama exist. Nadi Shuddhi Pranayama is the simplest. If performed along with Jal Neti and Jal Dhoti is a sure cure for asthma and allergies.
Prana means life or oxygen. Ayama means control. This process ensures **maximization of the use of oxygen** that is inhaled.

A] Anulom-vilom or nadi Shuddhi Pranayam B] Kapalbhati 3] Bhramari 4] Bhasarika, 5] Ujjayi 6] Agnisaar 7] Uddiyan bandha 8] Pranayam proper with fixed durations in set proportions for Rechaka [exhalation], Poorak [inhalation-2, Antar Kumbhak[Holding breath after Poorak]-3 and Rechaka-5. Bahya Kumbhak [optional-10]

Patanjali Kriya
Hath yoga includes all of the above practices and Shuddhi Kriya.
Gyan yoga means Dhyan and Dharana.
Note – Each asana or Kriya should be performed with total focus on the sensations that arise in the body. Every movement should be easy and slow and with a flow. Every feeling should be full of happiness.

DHYAN AND DHARANA

Mindfulness Meditation is the term coined by Dr. Richard Davidson, Professor of Psychiatry, and Wisconsin University, USA. Author has termed BK-Rajayoga as Internal silence [Antar mauna] oriented mindfulness meditation.

BK- Rajayoga- Meditation

It has some similarities with Spiritually augmented Cognitive Behavioral Therapy [S.A.C.B.T.] which is the latest in Psychiatry for mind empowerment.

Brahma Kumaris Rajayoga technique as taught in 11500 BK-centres in 140 countries has the following essential components. Each component augments the beneficial effect of other components. Hence the technique is of paramount importance. [Vidhi se hi siddhi hai]. Miraculous benefits are obtained within three months if the technique is followed fully and totally. The schedule should form the total and **indispensible component of daily routine** of a practitioner to derive maximum benefits. This is the much needed lifestyle **modification** today.

Essential Components of BK- Lifestyle

A] **Amrit vela Meditation** at 4am to 5am regularly without break. This period of time is known in scriptures as Brahma muhurtha.

B] Traffic control- A **brief Meditation** for just one minute every one hour. This helps to restore elevated consciousness that is usually lost in the present atmosphere of gross negativity.

C] A brief meditation for ten to fifteen minutes before going to sleep. It wipes out the negative transcription of the mind and ensures a deep and refreshing sleep.

D] News Papers and TV serials give a constant and huge diet of toxic emotions. They should be avoided in the morning and two hours before going to sleep. Toxic emotions and negative thoughts deplete Prana or Life Force Energy. Both of them initiate a subtle onslaught of Free radicals or Terror molecules on Longevity genes. This results in **early ageing**, cataracts and heart attacks.

E] Satvik Paushtik vegetarian food is essential but not compulsory. Food should be prepared and eaten in a happy atmosphere and in remembrance of God. Whole focus [Mindfulness] should be on food and on the act of eating. Thus watching TV serial during eating is strictly prohibited. But for the modern man with TV-addiction this may be difficult. **Mind control by meditation shall help you.**

F] Satsang- Daily visit to a BK centre for listening to Celestial **Murali is considered as the food for the soul or Atman.**-

Murali is a Divine four page script that gives a regular input of **powerfully positive** and motivating thoughts from **Supreme Soul** [Param Atma].The **miraculous mind empowerment** by this simple ritual has to be **personally experienced to be believed. Dr. Naras Bhat ,USA**, in his excellent book entitled Stress Physiology quotes that any positive thought repeated for sizeable duration[may be half an hour or more] for **21 days** is embedded deeply in psyche and brings about a positive behavioral change. No wonder **the figure 21 chosen by Shri Ganesh is very auspicious.**

One can access the Muralis on internet or by watching 24 hours Peace of Mind channel on TV.

TRAFFIC CONTROL
A BRIEF ONE MINUTE MEDITATION EVERY ONE HOUR OR SO

Bring your consciousness to get focused in the centre of the forehead, in between the two eye brows. This is the site for **Agya Energy Chakra**. This is also the site for the Third eye or a spiritual eye. So Har har Mahadeva means each one of us has a **Third eye**. When it opens in Divine guidance during meditation, all of our negativity gets burnt out.

A single auto suggestion needs to be repeated for the whole one minute-

"I am a peaceful soul. I am a loveful soul, blissful soul, pure soul or powerful soul. I am a soul and I am not this body. I am the metaphysical conscient point of light situated at Agya chakra."

The technique involves visualizing each particular quality of the soul and **dwelling in its "Experience"** for some time. This "Experience" then gets imbibed into your psyche or subconscious mind. This implant of a seed of a thought sprouts automatically when the circumstances require that particular quality. Eg. In an encounter with a troublesome person the qualities of peace, power and compassion get emerged. Soon it has a tranquilizing effect on that troubled soul and the situation is saved. Russian R & D institutes attribute this effect to thought vibrations emanating from the soul of a Sadhak [practitioner].

Human mind is experiential. All of its permanent learning happens by acquiring "Experience." Spiritual knowledge is the conglomerate of "Collective Experiences" and "Mystical experiences [Sakshatkars]" of highly enlightened and evolved souls.

LONG VERSION- RAJAYOGA MINDFULNESS BASED STRESS REDUCTION PROGRAMME [R-M.B.S.R.P.]

MEDITATION DONE AT AMRUT VELA [4am for one hour]

PREAMBLE-

The place fixed for meditation should be the same every day. A pure and powerful atmosphere is created around that place by powerful positive thoughts emanating from Atman during meditation.

Sit comfortably with a straight back on a chair. Sukhasana or Padmasan postures on a mat are the best. This posture keeps the **seven energy** chakras of the body in same alignment. This ensures a free **flow of cosmic energy** through seven energy chakras from the top to bottom- Sahasara, Agya, Vishuddhi, Anahat, Manipura, Swadhishthan and Muladhar chakra. These energy chakras are actually the distribution points [D.P.] for **life-force energy** [Prana]. The flow of cosmic energy is called as Cosmic Vibrational Healing Whisper by Dr. Naras Bhat, a cardiologist and a Mind Body Medicine Specialist in USA. Now perform abdominal type of breathing ten times. This process helps to calm down

R-M.B.S.R.P. involves following techniques:-
A] **Cyber scan** of own thoughts
B] **Heart felt Resonance Imaging [H.R.I.]**- shows the predominant thought or thoughts occupying one's mind and reveals the "Experience" or sensations one's Self or Atman is getting from such thoughts. Vipassana, Buddhist form of Meditation by Lord Gautama Buddha calls this process as "Differential perception." A negative thought or emotion always creates a bad feeling or sensation. Predominant thought forms a Primary Motivational Factor [P.M.F.]for the Atman. Therefore **Bhagavad Gita** tells us that a thought form the seed of our karma and destiny.
C] Auto-suggestions or self-hypnosis
D] Visualization or guided imagery.

E] STEPS OF LONG VERSION MEDITATION

1. Focus
2. Internalization
3. Cosmic Communion.
4. Post Meditation Suggestions [PMS]

First step-   Focus- Bahya Tratak-

Repeat each of the autosuggestions ten times. Visualize whatever words are spoken in the commentary.eg. I am an Ananda swaroop soul. Visualize the moment when you were full of happiness.

A] Give an auto-suggestion number one- I am a soul. **I am not this body.**

I the soul am a metaphysical conscient point of light which is immortal, indestructible and diseaseless. I a conscient of point of light am situated in the centre of the forehead in between two eye brows..

I am a peaceful, loveful, blissful, powerful and **pure** soul.

Purity has three levels-

1] Brahmacharya Celibacy- This is the purity at the level of body consciousness. It is required in **Balya Avastha** or learning phase of life. Our own research [Aurangabad] has proved that chewing five leaves of **Neem** daily helps to achieve celibacy.

Grihasthashram is governed by the rules pertaining to it.

Vanaprastha avastha means a process of withdrawing our consciousness from the external to the internal world. This is an inner **ever blissful voyage** into the fourth dimension- spiritual dimension.

Sanyas- means developing such ruling and controlling power over one's mind that the temptations, attractions and pressures of the external world fail to affect us. This is the state of spiritual equilibrium **[Sthit-pragnya avastha]**. Dadi Janaki , the 100 years old Head of the Brahma kumaris has been certified by neurologists as the most stable mind in the whole world.

2] Purity at the level of thought- Ruling and controlling power over the mind is so powerful that not even one impure thought for any soul arises in the mind.

3] Highest level of purity- when you constantly have only the thoughts about the welfare of all the other persons or animals coming in contact with you. **[Shubh chintan and Shubh chintak]**

Note- A stage may come by the repeated autosuggestions when you shall lose all of the body consciousness and may "Experience" a belief that you a mere conscient point of light. However, achieving this stage requires a very long spiritual effort. But it is also true that till such a **body less state [Ashariri avastha]** is achieved by the consciousness a lifestyle following **Straight Path or Sirat al Mustaqim** takes care of your health, wealth, mental peace and happiness.

B] Now turn your attention to your thoughts.
They usually are running like superfast train in men with very high I.Q. today.
Give autosuggestion for ten times that the speed of thought is getting slower and slower.

C] Now turn your attention to your consciousness-
Perform a detail **Cyberscan** of your thoughts and categorize them into negative and waste thoughts, toxic emotions, positive thoughts and positive emotions. A rough percentage of positive and negative thoughts at this point time shall help to judge your progress and effect of spiritual effort. Perform **HRI-Heartfelt Resonance Imaging** to decide about the most predominant negative thought/emotion in your mind.
Give autosuggestion-   Let go .Don't get attached to thoughts. The speed of thoughts is gradually reducing.
Now turn your attention to your consciousness [Energy plus awareness].It is scattered like a diffuse sunlight. So it is ineffective.

Give autosuggestion-   My consciousness is getting focused on me, the conscient point of light in the centre of the forehead. Soon a single pointed focused state of consciousness shall be obtained.

As the focus increases the speed of thoughts shall get proportionately reduced. You shall be able to distinguish between the positive, negative and the waste thoughts as well as toxic emotions.[Daniel

Goleman]. Desires, Toxic emotions, negative thoughts and waste thought are responsible for the depletion of your pranik strength [Life Force].

Give autosuggestion-   All of my desires, toxic emotions, negative thoughts and waste thoughts are getting burnt out in the intense fire of my meditation [Yogagni].All of this negativity of mind is getting permanently deleted from my mind's computer.
A stage shall come when all the negativity shall get deleted from the mind's computer for one particular moment. When this happens, internalization of the consciousness takes place.

SECOND STEP OF R-MBSRP-   Internalization
Internalization of consciousness is indicated by a feeling of totally relaxed states of mind and body with a state of bliss. Dr. Herbert Benson, an American cardiologist who founded the first Institute of Mind and Body Medicine in 1970, uses two terms for denoting these states-
1] Biological Relaxation Response **BRR** [Shavasana] and
2] The zone.**[Ekagra Chitta Avastha].**

This state of consciousness, a soul conscious or Satvik state is very important.
1] Various autosuggestions become most powerful and effective in this state.
2] Rejuvenating neuro hormones FROM THE BRAIN are secreted in this state.

3] Delta waves of deep sleep pattern are recorded usually after a regular practice [sadhana] of 2 years.

4] Lactic acid giving tiredness is quickly metabolized.

5] Secretion of stress hormones and free radicals stops.

6] Potentiation of immune system happens giving a quantum jump in resistance to infections, cancer cells, allergens and auto-antigens.

7] A quantum Jump in self-determination [Will power], Quality of Life [QOL] and E.E.H. value of life [Energy, Enthusiasm and happiness] happens.

Proof of the pudding lies in tasting it. This is known as "Experiential evidence" which has been in use for tasting the effectiveness of medicinal herbs in Ayurveda. The need for expensive state of art equipment to demonstrate an "Experience" by the practitioner of Yog- Transcendental experience." becomes redundant. One can discover whole of God instead of one God's particle if one has belief and faith.

Medical wing of Brahma kumaris [R.E.R.F.- Rajayoga Education and Research Foundation]has some novel instruments- 1] Thought graph machine [in S.P.A.R.C. wing], 2] Aura scanner 3] Happiness index machine and 4] RespErate . However, these instruments require scientific validation by recognized research institutes.

Some Prototypes of disease-specific autosuggestions

1] Anger management- My anger and irritation has disappeared permanently from my mind's computer. I always remember that I am a peaceful, loveful and blissful soul.

2] Stress management- I am a peaceful, loveful and powerful soul. So the stress, tension, anxiety, worry fear or frustration can never contaminate my Satvik consciousness.

3] R-MBSRT for the prevention and cure of the cancer-
One cancer cell is formed after each 10 raised to 17 cell divisions. Natural Killer cells [NK-cells] are the James Bond of the body. They quickly identify and destroy the cancer cell that has been formed. Hence most of us are cancer free till the last breath. So these autosuggestions may prevent cancer.

Autosuggestion and visualization for prevention and cure of cancer-
A cosmic energy, a cosmic healing Vibrational healing whisper is entering my body through the top most Sahasara energy chakra and passing through all the subsequent energy chakras – Agya, Vishuddhi, Anahat, Manipura, Swadhishthan and Muladhar chakra and bringing a rejuvenation. The fire of meditation is so intense that this cosmic energy is burning out each and every cancer cell in my body. NK-cells in my body are quickly discovering the newly formed cancer cells and destroying them. Thus I am attaining a cancer free state.

4] For De-addiction programme-
All of the addictions happen because of stress after stress, lack of mental peace and happiness in life. So the autosuggestions focus on mental peace and happiness.

Autosuggestion -1- I am a peaceful, loveful and blissful soul. I am so powerful that I can easily resist the urge to drink or smoke for getting a temporary "High".

Autosuggestion-2- The neuro-hormones, DHEA, endorphins and Anandamide are natural and most powerful pain killers and mood elevators. So my feeling of unhappiness is disappearing from my mind. The sense of feeling good is so powerful that I shall never indulge in my addiction which gives only a temporary "High."

5] Performance enhancement-
As the Scientist Mind achieves silence [Antar-mauna] lateral thinking or Out Of Box thinking begins. This is responsible for intuition [gut feeling or sixth sense] which enhances the power of split second best decision for the problem solving. The suggestion comes to the mind in a split second as if from cosmos. Creativity of the mind is enhanced which could be of great help in innovation. Artists may create such supreme designs or painting which may appear beyond the scope of human thinking. A man can achieve anything if he has a mind to do it.

Third step of R-MBSRP - Cosmic Communion

Visualization or guided imagery plays a great role in this step.

Visualize that I, the soul, a conscient point of light have come out of my body of five elements and undertaken a cosmic travel to Supreme abode [Param Dham] of all the souls. All of us are mere guests on this planet earth. We descend on the planet earth in the costume or body to play our respective roles in a huge world drama. The costume, the type of life and the role are decided by our past karmic accounts. Good karmic account means happiness, health and harmony. Bad karmic account means diseases, defects, early deaths, accidents, pain and suffering. A human being thus always has two choices in life. Right choice means happy and healthy life.

I am now travelling through the world of stars, moon and the sun. I have now arrived in the Micro-world of the Trinity- Brahma, the Creator and Governor, Vishnu the operator and Mahesh the Destroyer. Mahesh destroys the negativity in my mind. I now enter into Param Dham after taking the blessings from the Trinity.

In Param Dham I am experiencing a joy and peace that is beyond words. I am surrounded by a reddish yellow rejuvenating light. I am now standing in front of God, Shiva, Shiva baba, Who is Supreme Father of all the souls, Supreme teacher and Supreme Sadgatidata data. He is also a Conscient Point of Light and incorporeal. He is a Point in appearance but an ocean of peace, happiness, power and of everything one desires in life. I am His beloved son/daughter. So whatever He has, I have a birth right over it. Red rays of power and white rays of peace and purity are emanating from the Supreme Soul [Param-Atma].I am imbibing theses rays and becoming more powerful and peaceful.

Visualize this scene for quite some time.

Visualize that I am getting richer and richer in eights powers that are necessary in life. The power of tolerance is most essential. But if while tolerating one gets a constant feeling that only "I" am tolerating and suffering then it is not true tolerance. Cosmic Universal laws tell that acquiring one power attracts other powers as if from Cosmos. Power of judgment and right decision is another very important power of the soul. An "Inner voice" always shouts loudly when a man is about to commit wrong. The right or wrong is decided by eternal cosmic laws. Enhanced power of judgment is necessary for the best solutions to the problems in life. Power of accommodation, co-operation, condensation and power to face and finish are other important powers one acquires in cosmic communion with Supreme Father.

Now I after getting enriched with power and peace I am undertaking the return journey. I have crossed the Micro-world of Trinity and also the world of Sun, Moon and stars. Now I have come to rest on my eternal seat in between the two eye brows.

Visualize- The rays and vibrations of power, peace, purity, love and bliss are spreading through each and every cell of the body rejuvenating and re-charging them. Dwell in this "Experience" for some time.

Post Meditation Suggestions

Now give two auto suggestions to the mind-

1] Let me remain in this elevated powerful soul conscious state throughout the day while performing my tasks under any circumstances which may try to disturb this state of consciousness.

2] Next day, at 4am, Amrit –vela when I begin my meditation [yog with Supreme Soul] let me begin from this elevated state of consciousness so that with each day I shall become more powerful, peaceful, loveful, blissful and pure.

REFERENCES

1.   Naras Bhat- Reversing stress and burn out. 2002. Cybernetix Publishing.2182, East Street, Concord, California   94520,   USA.   Email- StressBook@heartsaver.com

2.   Naras Bhat- How to reverse and prevent Heart disease and cancer? 1995. Dr. Kumar Pati at New Editions   Publishing1675   Rollins   Road,   Suit B3,Burlingame, California 94010 phone [415]697-4400 Fax-[415]697-7937

3.   Marshall Govindan- Kriya yoga Sutras of Patanjali and the Siddhas. Translation, Commentary and practice. 2000. Babaji's Kriya Yoga Order of Acharyas Trust.   Post   Box-   5608,   Malleshweram   West, Bengaluru.560055. email - kriyayog@vsnl.com

4.   Satish K. Gupta, Ramesh C. Sawhney, Lajapt Rai, V.D. Chavan, Sameer Dani, Ramesh C. Arora,, V. Selvamurthy, H.K. Chopra,, Navin C. Nanda- Regression of coronary atherosclerosis through healthy lifestyle in coronary artery disease patients- Mount Abu Open Heart Trial. Indian Heart J. 2011;63;461-469

5.   S.D. Kaundinya, D.V. Kaundinya: - Meditation versus   relaxation-   A   comprehensive   review- International J. of Basic and Applied Physiology. Vol-2,p- 240-257;December 2013

6.   D.V. Kaundinya – Brahma Kumaris Rajayoga- An evidence based internal silence oriented meditation as cure for the incurable and chronic diseases[NCD] and addictions. International J. of Current Medicine And Applied Sciences. July 2014

APPENDIX - II

Pranayam Motivated Defaecation

A recent survey has shown that 14% of all Indians including the young suffer from mild to severe constipation. Severe constipation is very common in senior age group or the patients in Geriatric O.P.D. Several have to take enema on regular basis. Some have an experience of taking out the faecal nuggets with fingers. Lack of exercise, Pizza Burger Cola diet and Non-vegetarian diet are some of the important contributing factors. Over use of Over The Counter [OTC] pills or purgatives weaken the walls of intestine. Shortly it results in weak peristalsis or propelling movement of the intestine.

Hydrotherapy prior to P.M.D. Programme-
Warning- Never strain while defecating if you wish to avoid piles or fissures. Everything in yogic practices is done with ease.

Prior hydrotherapy- It is necessary to hydrate oneself well one day prior to P.M.D. Drink a minimum of 15 to 20 glasses of water throughout the day. It is necessary to drink water even if one is not thirsty. This is because with advancing age, the reflex initiating the drinking process gets progressively weaker. **The test for adequate hydration is that the urine always remains clear like water.** Henceforth make it a practice to drink plenty of water throughout your life.

Jal Dhauti is a yogic kriya if performed for one month ensures adequate hydration and effective purging out of accumulated toxins.

Take four to five glasses of water or more if you can, no sooner one gets up at 4am.[Amrit-vela]. Warm water with a pinch of salt is helpful initially. A session of Pranayam after Amrit-vela meditation should be followed by P.M.D. Isabgol at night may help but required only initially. Learning Shuddhi kriyas like Jal Dhauti and Pranayam called Agnisaar helps.

Relaxation of mind by meditation plays a significant role. Never sing – Tu atki hai kanha, main tadapata yanha. This creates a negative programming of your mind. Instead sing. ,"Chal akela chal akela, Tera maila peeche chchuta, tu chal akela. This shall be a positive programming of your mind for the task at hand.

Do not contaminate the elevated Satvik consciousness achieved by meditation by taking a newspaper or your problems to the toilet seat. Focus your attention on your colon. Here the single pointed focus achieved by meditation helps greatly. Visualize about a faecal bolus stuck up at the appendix side of the colon. Now breathing deeply [abdominal breathing] visualize that the bolus is gradually getting unstuck. Now it is moving forward with each progressive contraction of the colon. Agnisaar at this point of time helps. Visualize that the bolus is now travelling in the ascending colon. Now it has entered the Transverse colon. Its forward movement has now become quicker. Visualize that now the bolus has entered descending colon and speedily going to the end of the rectum. Now a final push and it is out of the body. Do not strain at this point of time as it may cause piles to form. Each process has to be done with ease without straining at any point. Immense relief and joy at this point of time is beyond words. In fact you shall also see the relief writ large on the faces of the people around you, especially in an elevator.

Within a month you shall be colon trained and defecation shall be as easy as taking a breath.

BK- Rajayoga restores the SNS Versus PNS balance [Sympathetic Nervous System and Parasympathetic Nervous System] which is usually disturbed in Diabetes. This is the common cause of constipation in Diabetics.

Disturbed Internal balance of ions, sugar and lipids also contribute to N.C.D.s like Head ache, Migraine, Acidity, High B.P., Diabetes and Heart attacks.

Gut Like Protein –I and II released from Gastro intestinal tract helps in controlling appetite in Diabetes.

Medical science behind each and every ancient yogic practice needs to be investigated by a systematic research in Medical Institutes. There is a paucity of this type of research because the Indians themselves have stopped believing in the ancient Indian spiritual wisdom. Whole of the world is engaged in yog while Indians are pursuing the lifestyle of Bhog and Rog.

09-10-2017

BK Dr. Dilip V. Kaundinya